# Erotic Massage

## Now Available In Video!

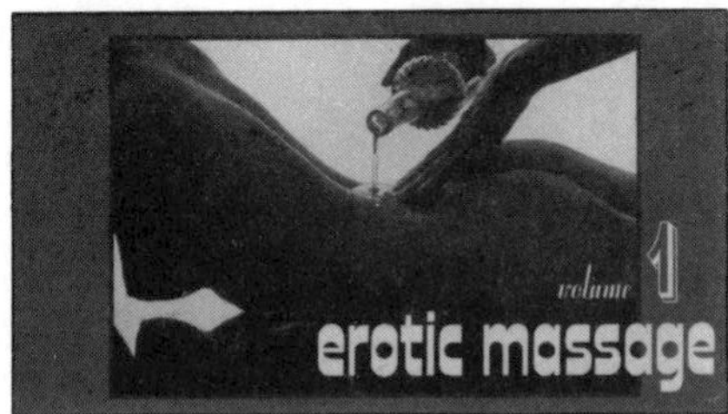


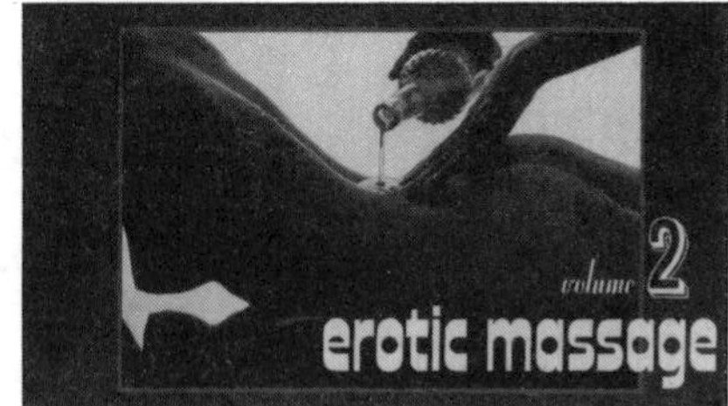


Designed to complement the step-by-step instruction in this book, the educational videos demonstrate the gentleness, the respect, the grace of the strokes integrated into a total experience. In easy-to-learn strokes, you and your partner can bring together the sensual, the erotic, and the intimate.

***NOTICE: This is an explicit, two-volume video. Nudity and genital massage are shown. What you will see is sensitive, caring massage for the whole body in the privacy of your home.***

**VOLUME ONE:** the back, the feet, the neck, the face, and more—all the strokes in the book except the genital massage, in the same order as in the book.

**VOLUME TWO:** the female and male genital massage as in the book, plus new, unwritten strokes.

For Private Home Use Only.
VHS / Hi-Fi Stereo / Color / 30 Minutes Each Volume

Also Available from Secret Garden Publishing • www.SecretGardenPublishing.com

BOOKS • by Kenneth Ray Stubbs, Ph.D. • DVDs and Videos

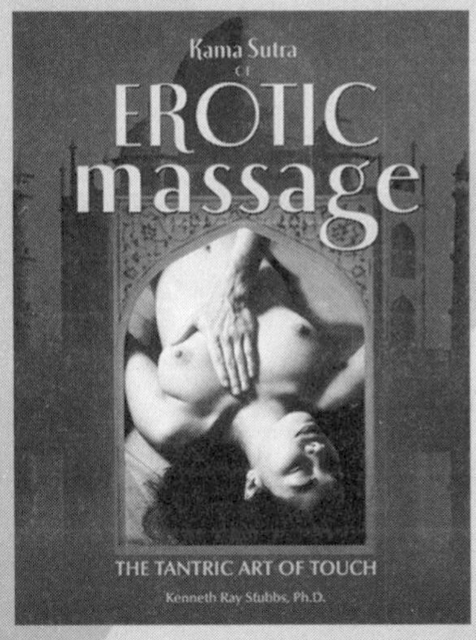


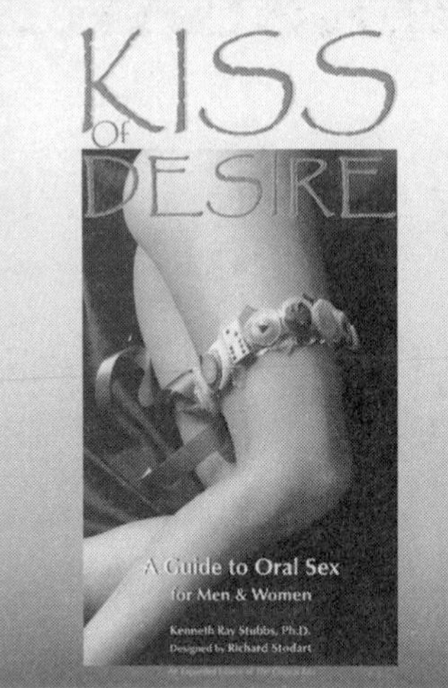


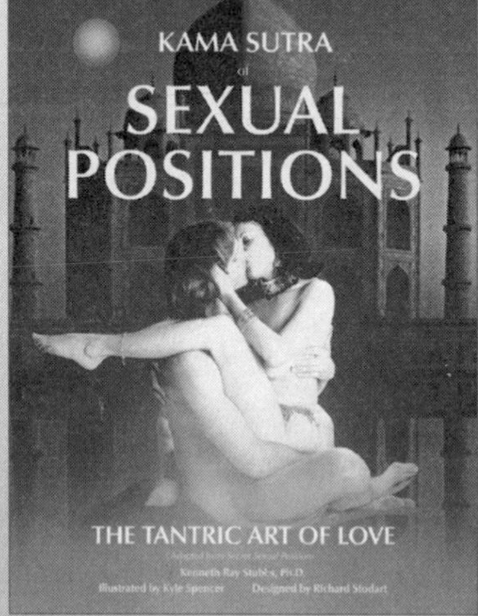


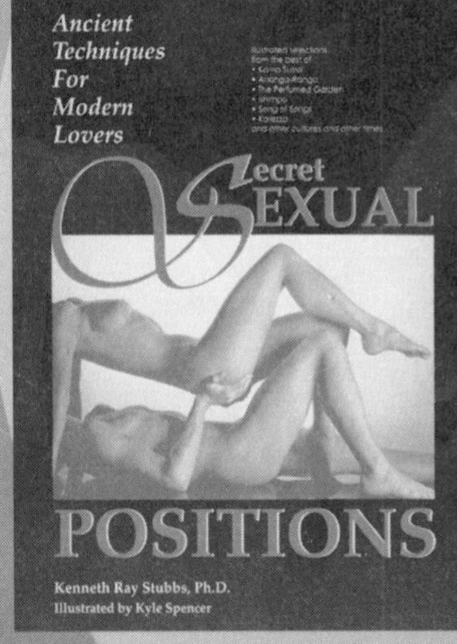


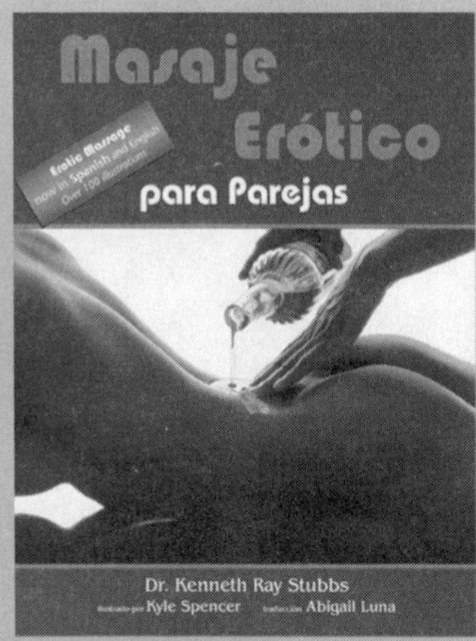


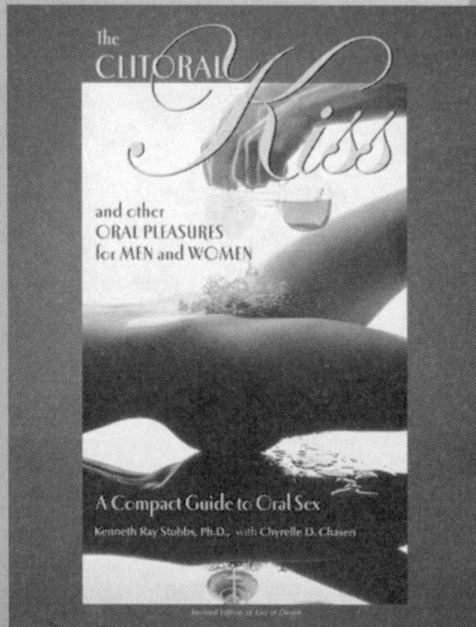


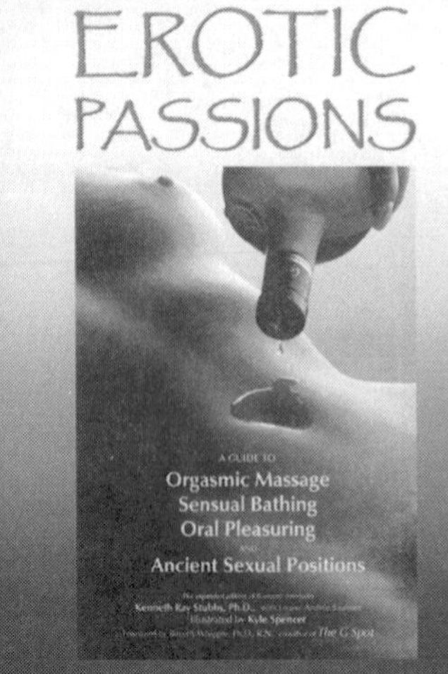


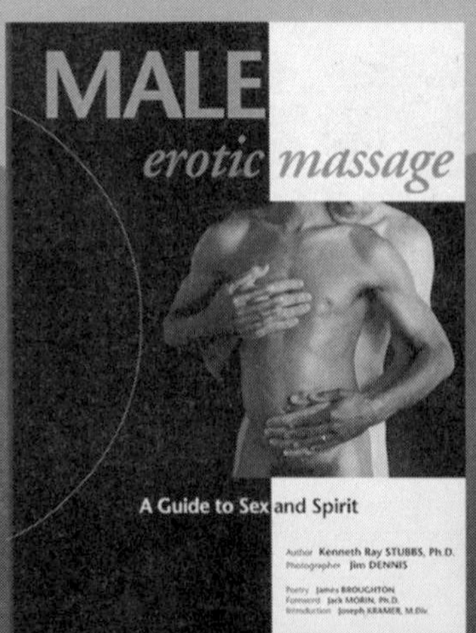


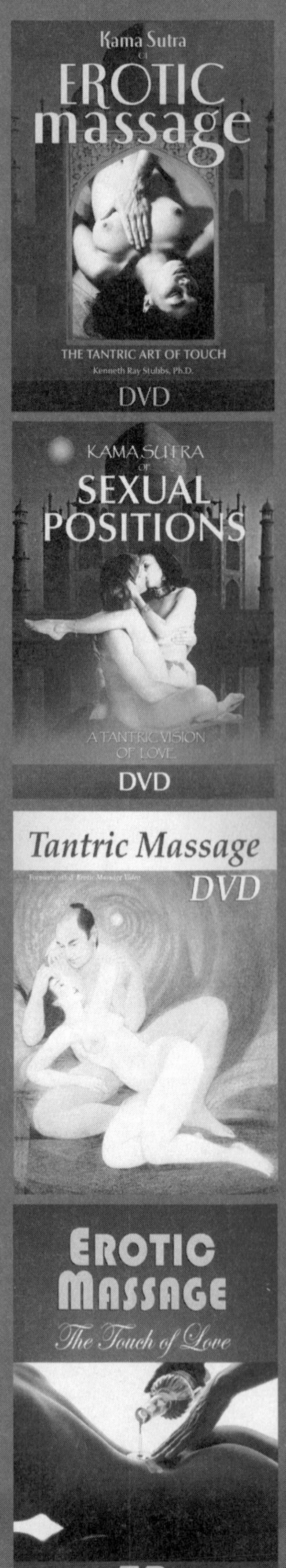

# EROTIC MASSAGE

## THE TOUCH OF LOVE

An Illustrated, Step-by-Step Manual for Couples

by

Kenneth Ray Stubbs, Ph.D.
with
Louise-Andrée Saulnier

Illustrated
by
Kyle Spencer

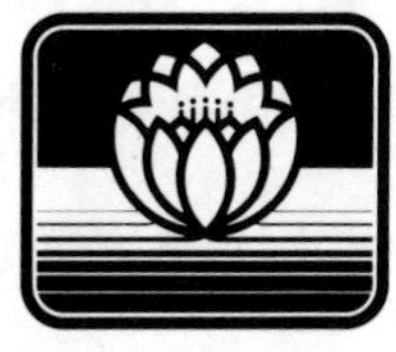

Secret Garden

Published by **Secret Garden Publishing**
5631 W. Placita del Risco
Dept. BEM
Tucson, AZ 85745

**www.SecretGardenPublishing.com**


Printed in the United States of America

Illustrations: Kyle Spencer
Based on photography by Ellen Gunther
Front Cover Photo: David Thorpe
Back Cover Photo: Flavio Amorin

ISBN 0-939263-02-5

40 39 38 37 36 35 34 33 32 31 30 29 28 27 26

❧ ❧ ❧

**A Word of Caution**

The purpose of this book is to educate. It is not intended to give medical or psychological therapy. Whenever there is concern about physical or emotional illness, a qualified professional should be consulted.

The authors, illustrator, and publisher shall have neither liability nor responsibility to any person or entity with respect to any loss, damage, injury, or ailment caused or alleged to be caused directly or indirectly by the information or lack of information in this book.

❧ ❧ ❧

# RECOMMENDATION

**LAY THE BOOK FLAT**
**TO LEARN THE STROKES**

1. Take Erotic Massage to a "fast print" shop.
2. For a few dollars, have the shop
   a. cut off the binding,
   b. punch comb binding holes near the binding edge,
   c. and place a comb binding on the edge.

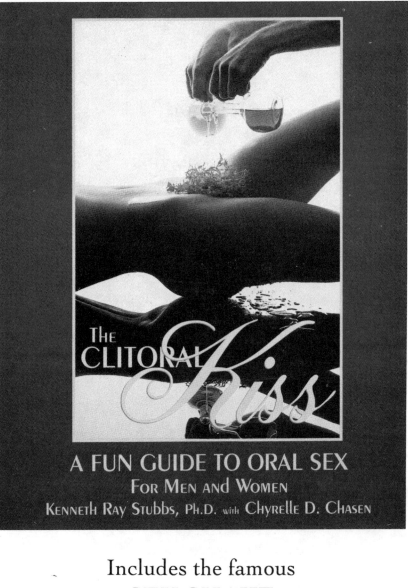

Dedicated to

Suzanne Myers
and
Paul Fleming

Your gifts are remembered.

# CONTENTS

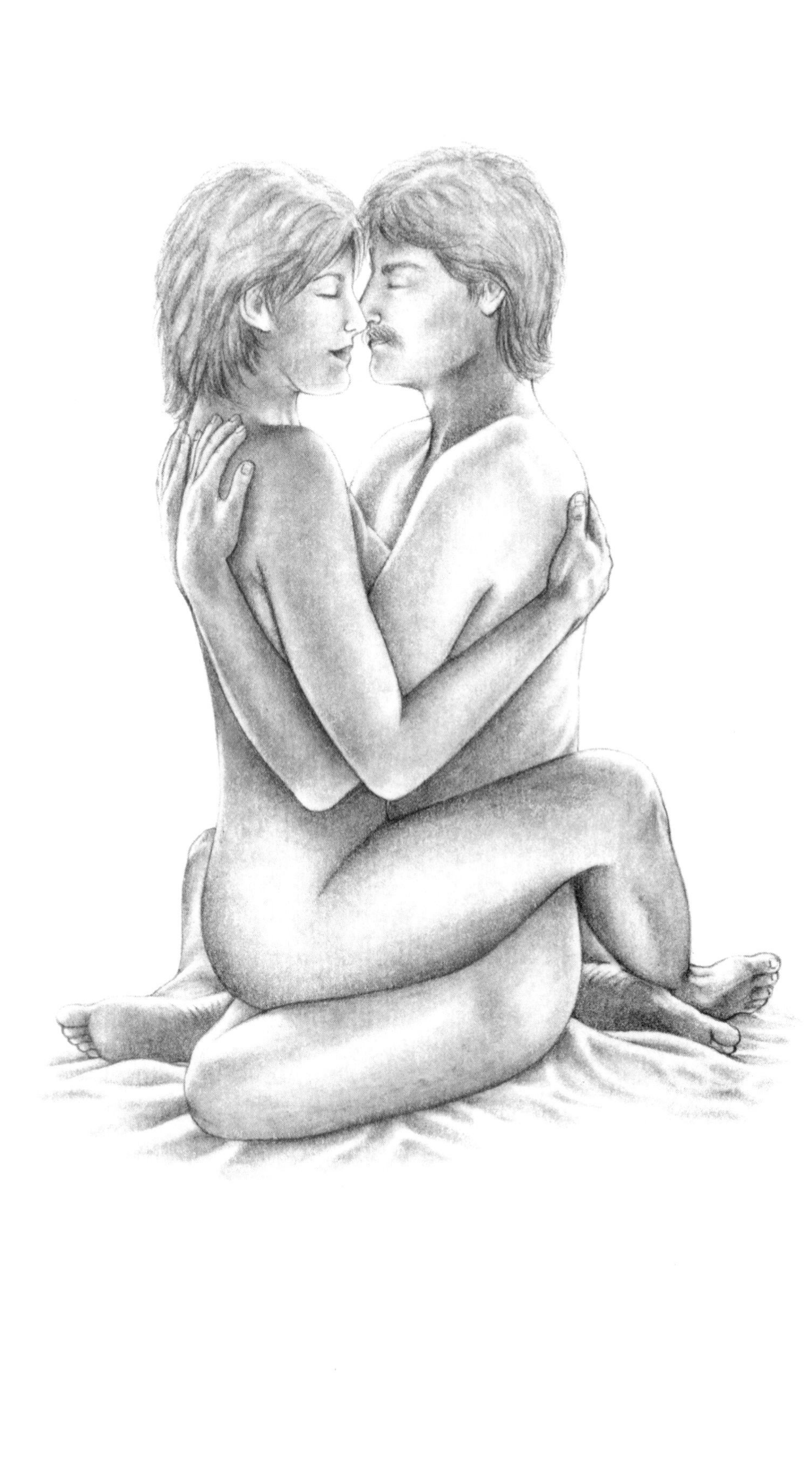

# INVITATION

This is a language
without words.

This is a time
outside of time.

This is a song
that sings
a celebration.

This is the touch of love.

# INTRODUCTION

This is a book about love.

Love
is a feeling.

To express love
is called
nurturing.

This is a love book especially for lovers.
Your boyfriend, your girlfriend
your wife
your husband
your significant other, your lover, your mate
the label is not important
the feeling is.

You may be friends
exploring becoming lovers.

You may be lovers
exploring becoming friends.

What is most important
is that
what you do
is
consensual.

Massage simply stated
simply is
patterned touch.
We might say
a caress
is unpatterned touch.
Which you choose to give
or to receive
depends on the mood.
Be open to either.
Both heal.
Both nurture.
Both excite.

During the massage,
either or both of you
might feel erotic.
You might fall asleep.
You might burst out in laughter
or in tears.

You might or might not
have sex before,
during,
or after.
However, should sex or orgasm become
the goal,
you might miss
many other pleasures.

Allow each moment
each feeling
to unfold
itself.

# Introduction

Massage
is an art
when you
express yourself
    with sensitivity
    with awareness.

Let your touch
discover
    without demands
    without expectations.

At first
the techniques
will be
techniques,
like learning
to ride a bicycle.
After a while
the awkward will become
familiar.

Your touch
will come
to nourish
the body
the mind
and
the spirit.

You will also find
your lover's body
— in stillness —
pleasuring your hands.
Let your fingertips
taste
the curve
the rough, the smooth
the firm
the soft.

Let yourself feel.

# WHAT YOU NEED

A willing recipient

A quiet place

A warm place
or if it is tropical,
gentle breezes

Oil, perhaps a lotion—
on membranous tissue,
a water-based lubricant
may be healthier

A towel

A padded table
a bed or padded floor
or a large towel
on the beach

Soft music, if you wish

Perhaps
feathers, fur mitts
a silk scarf

# MASSAGE GUIDELINES

Three basic ones:

First and foremost,
be present.
Letting go of expectations
of the future
and
comparisons with the past,
Be
Here
Be
Now.

Secondly
maintain full-hand contact
whenever possible.
Allow your palms,
fingers,
and thumbs
to outline the contours.

Thirdly
maintain a continuous flow.
Movements blend together,
each one
enhancing the preceding one
and preparing the next.

More important
than the techniques
is
your own personal expression.

More important than
your own personal expression
is
the recipient's wishes.

More important than
the recipient's wishes
is
your never forcing yourself.
Yet
be open to discovering
new horizons.
It's a delicate balance.

# REMINDERS

If the sensation
feels good to the recipient,
you are doing it correctly,
regardless
of theory or written instructions.

Vary
the pressure,
the tempo,
the rhythm.
Repeating a stroke in the exact same way each time
becomes boring very quickly
to both the recipient and the giver.

If there are two of them,
massage both.

Glide on and off.
To begin a touch,
rather than plopping on,
glide on with a slow descent
in the direction
that your hands will be moving.
In coming off,
continue the movement in a gradual ascent.

Generally, minimize landings and takeoffs.

When in doubt,
lighter pressure might be better.
The recipient's preference, however,
is the best guide.
Ask occasionally, if you are uncertain.

Minimize the talking.
An important exception:
when the recipient needs
to communicate deep feelings.

Become centered.
Tuning into and slowing your breath,
you can quieten yourself.

Being centered,
you will experience more deeply
your own pleasure.

The following strokes assume
the massage is on a table.
Except for some of the long strokes,
most of the instructions can be adapted
to floor or bed massages.

Follow the presented sequence
or create a sequence
more suitable for your situation.

Massage the whole body
or only one section.

# HEALTH

Discussing health concerns
is essential
in establishing trust
in a relationship,
whether it be for an evening
or a lifetime.

If a partner has a cold or flu,
the other partner can choose
to be close
or not.

If there is an infectious condition on the skin,
forgo contact with that area.
Perhaps keep it clothed.

If there is a concern
about viral conditions
communicable through bodily fluids,
share your feelings with your partner.
Read this book's appendix,
*Eroticizing Safer-Sex.*
Consult agencies promoting healthy sex,
and read literature
which can assist you in choosing for yourself
what is best
in your sensual and sexual expressions.

Ask if there are any tender places.
Be especially gentle there
or exclude.
If an injury is severe
or if there are circulation problems,
first consult a health professional.

The debates continue
regarding the relative healthiness
of vegetable oil,
mineral oil,
and water-based lubricants
for massage on or in the body.
Many commercial preparations contain
preservatives, artificial colors,
and other chemical additives.
Some people are allergic
to added fragrances.
You may have to experiment first.

Regarding conception,
please make parenthood planned.

Now you are ready
to make the final preparations
for your special gift.

# PREPARATIONS

## Where?

Anywhere,
as long as distractions
and interruptions
are minimized.

Inside or outside is fine.
When outside,
take precautions for insects and excessive sun.
When inside,
unplug the phone.
Arrange for everyone else,
including children,
not to interrupt.

It is very important
to maintain a warm temperature.
If necessary, use a portable heater
or cover the areas of the body
you are not massaging at the moment.

## When?

Celebrate a birthday
an anniversary
Give a holiday-season present
handmade.

After intense work
during a stressful period.

Sometimes you can be spontaneous
but setting aside a specific day or evening
is more likely
to ensure it happening.

To give massage to a pregnant partner,
is a gift not forgotten.
In the later stages,
she may be unable to lie on her front or back.
Perhaps forgoe some strokes or positions,
but not the touch.

## With What?

Basically all you need is oil
    fragranced ones entice the mind
    but may sting the skin,
    especially membranous tissue.
Some prefer vegetable oils
(unfragranced coconut oil is a good choice)
others prefer mineral oils.
    Visit your local lotions-and-potions store,
    try a health food store.
On membranous tissues, such as the female genitals,
some consider water-based lubricants
to be healthier.
    Purchase them at a pharmacy,
    perhaps at a sensuous boutique.
You can apply the oil or lubricant to your hands
either from a plastic squeeze bottle,
a bottle with a push pump,
or a bowl.

Massage tables are great for your back,
and sturdy tabletops
padded with foam or blankets are fine.
Otherwise, a padded floor,
a bed,
or the ground covered with cloth
is quite suitable.

If you select a large bed,
have the recipient's head
at a corner of the foot of the bed
while his/her feet are pointing toward
the opposite corner at the head of the bed.
This will give you better access
to both the right and left sides.

For the covering cloth,
select a sheet or material
that is OK to be oiled.
Some fabrics are difficult to clean,
and the oily smell may not wash out.

Gather a large towel or two.

When lying on the front side,
the recipient may need a covered foam pad
or a couple of rolled towels
placed under the front of the ankles.

When lying on the back,
if there is strain in the lower back,
place the same pad underneath the knees.

If you anticipate using feathers
or other tactile stimulators,
have them close at hand.

Perhaps select some music
without dominating rhythms
without words — usually

Use candlelight or colored lights,
incense,
flowers,
interior design of the room,
or whatever creates a special ambience.
However,
you do not have to create Shangri-la every time.
Sometimes
all that is necessary
is
to close the door.

## Everything ready?

Oil,
phone unplugged,
temperature warm enough,
watches, jewelry, clothing removed,
recipient's contact lenses taken out (if necessary),
your finger nails smoothed,
your hands cleaned and warmed?

Ask if any strokes
on any particular places
would be particularly pleasing.

Ask for other possible relevancies
such as preferences for no oil in the hair
or time limitations.

Once your lover
is ready to begin,
give the invitation
to take a few fuller breaths
and
to close his/her eyes.

Allowing
your hands
to move intuitively,
you can open doors
to inner peace
to pleasure
to joy
    both your lover's
    and
    yours.

# THE MASSAGE

# BEGINNING

Lover's Position: Lying front down with arms by side.
Your Position: Initially at your lover's left side.

Laying On Of Hands

## 1. Laying On Of Hands

1. A

**A.**
**Center yourself.**
**Tune into your breathing.**

1. B

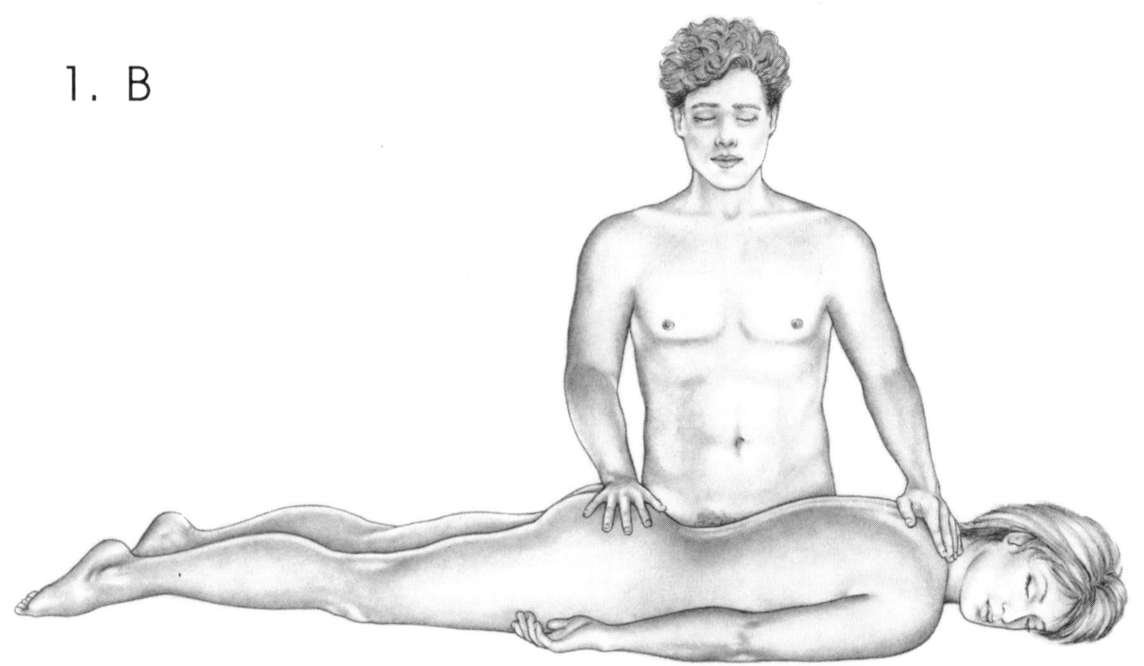

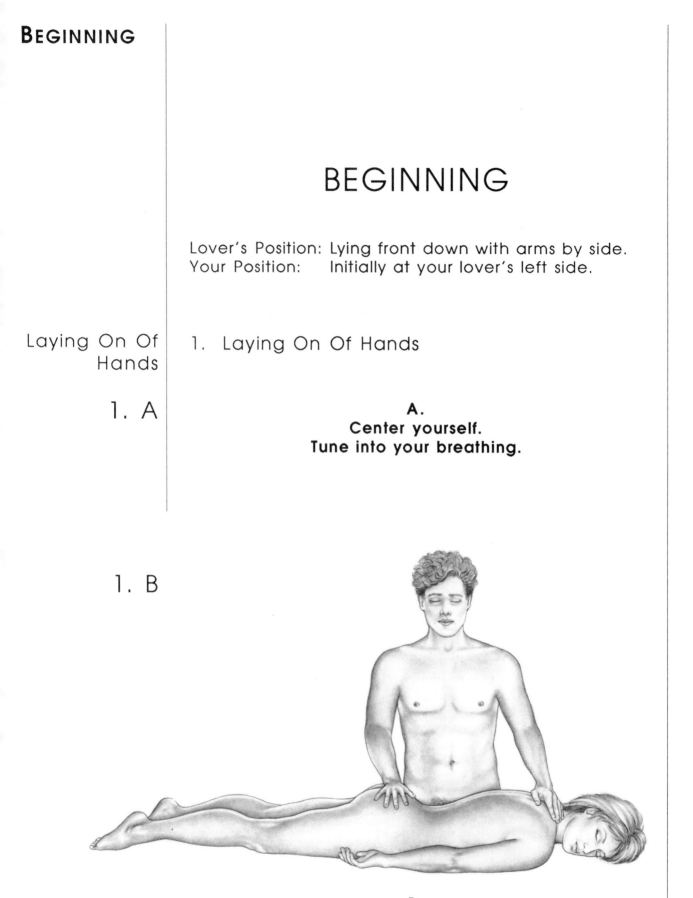

**B.**
**Rest your left palm on the upper back, your right palm on the sacrum.**

Laying On Of Hands

1. C

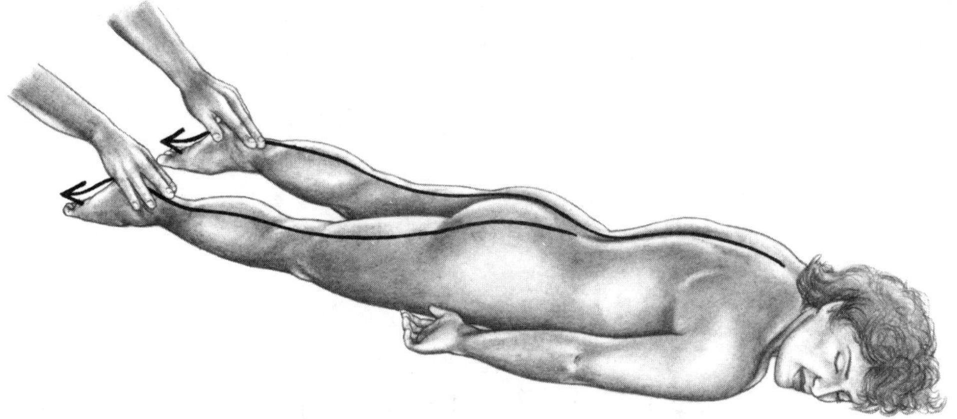

C.
Lightly pull your hands downward,
separating at the waist
and then flowing down off the tips of the toes.

If you have feathers, fur mitts,
or other sensuous materials,
stroke your lover
- all over -
now
*before* you apply any oil.

**Beginning**

Spreading Oil
2. A

2. B

## 2. Spreading Oil

**A.**
**Warm oil in your hands.**
**(Be careful not to let drops fall on your partner.)**

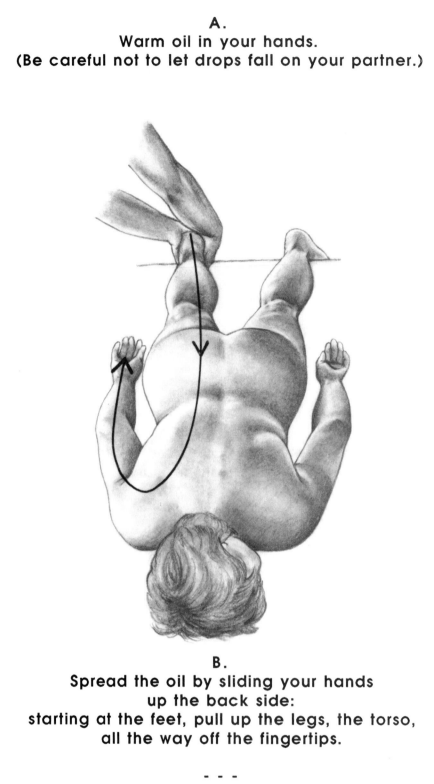

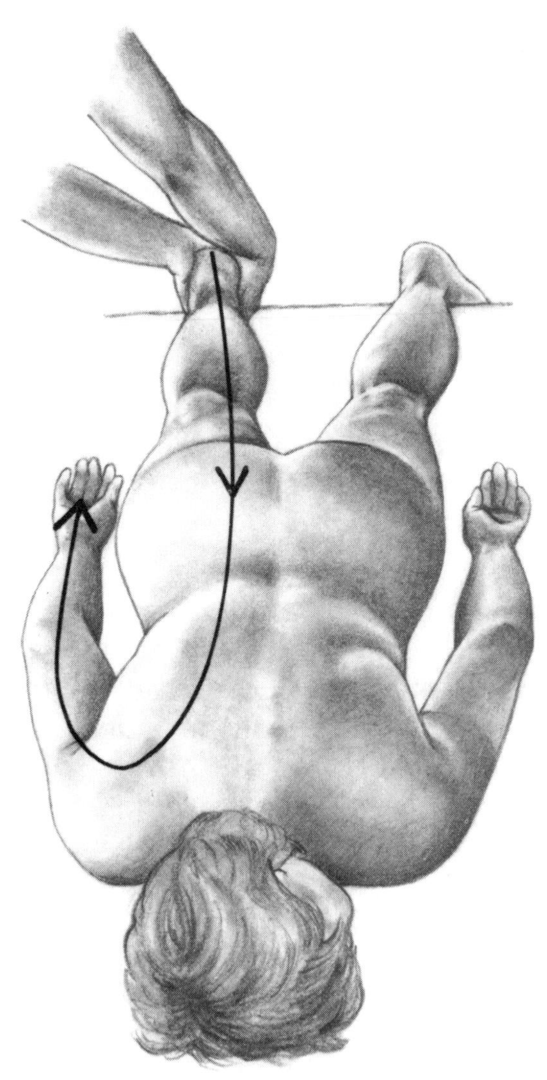

**B.**
**Spread the oil by sliding your hands up the back side:**
**starting at the feet, pull up the legs, the torso, all the way off the fingertips.**

\- - -

**Repeat the same sequence on the other side.**
**(It is easier if you first move to the other side.)**

**This is not the only oil application.**
**Generally, you add more oil in the initial stroke of each section.**

# BACK

Your Position: Initially at your lover's head and facing his/her feet.

## 3. Connecting Stroke

Connecting Stroke

3. A

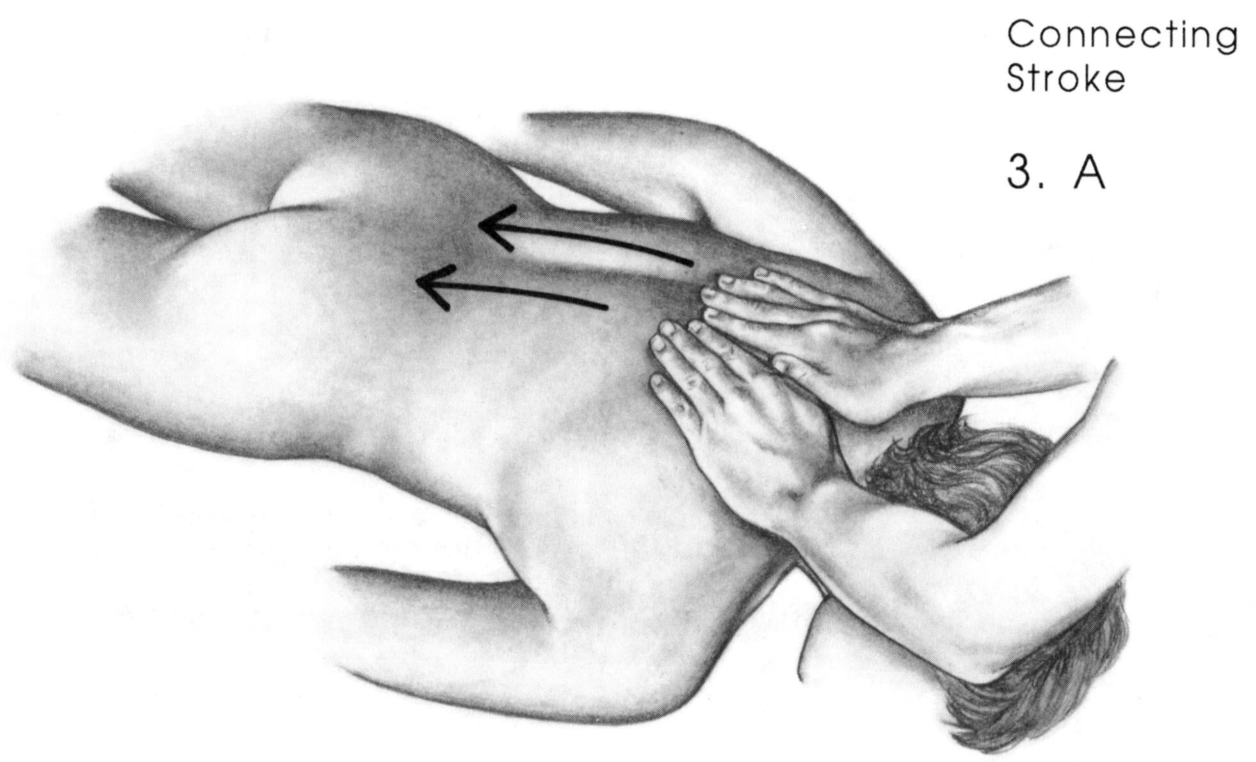

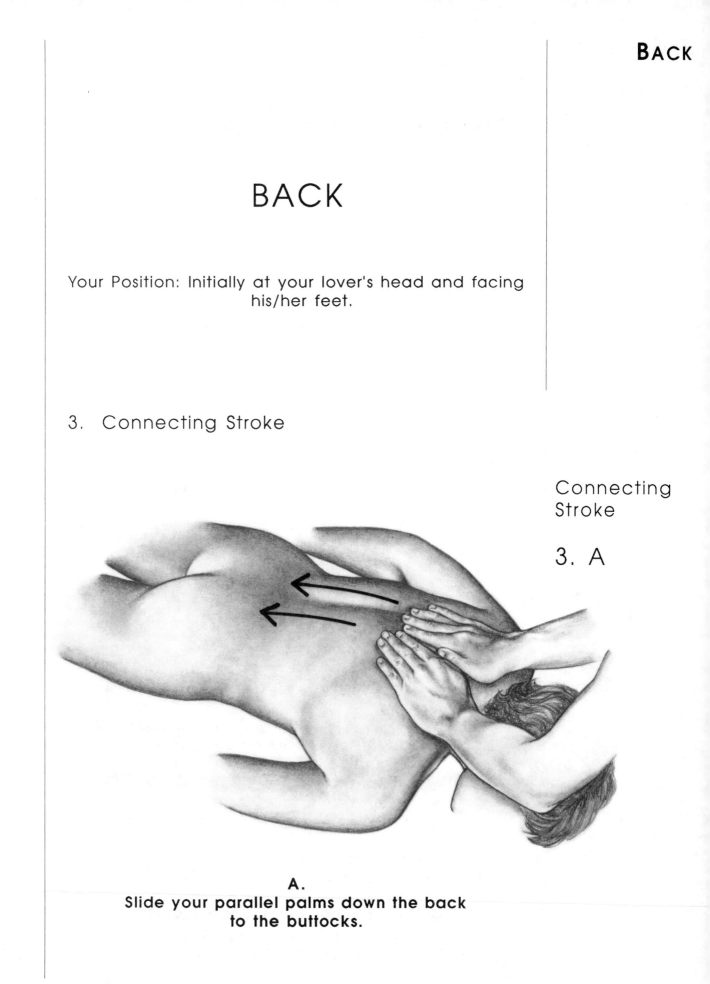

**A.**
**Slide your parallel palms down the back to the buttocks.**

Connecting Stroke

3. B

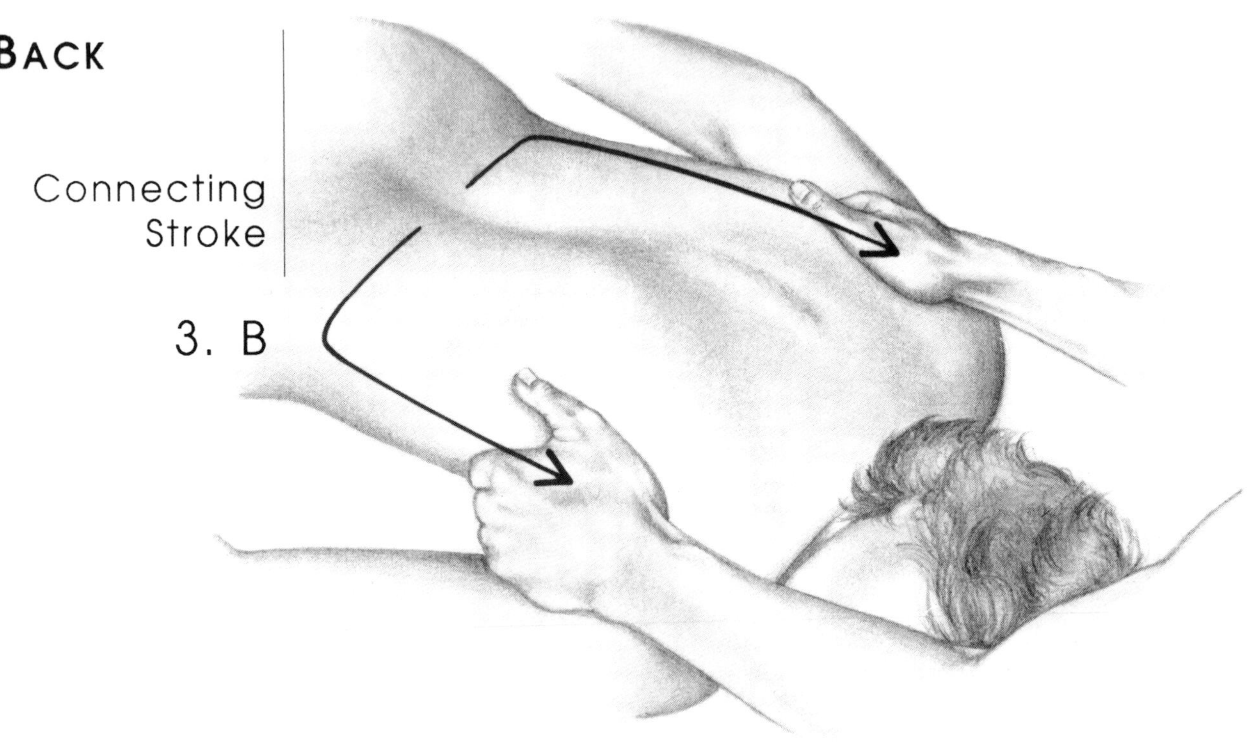

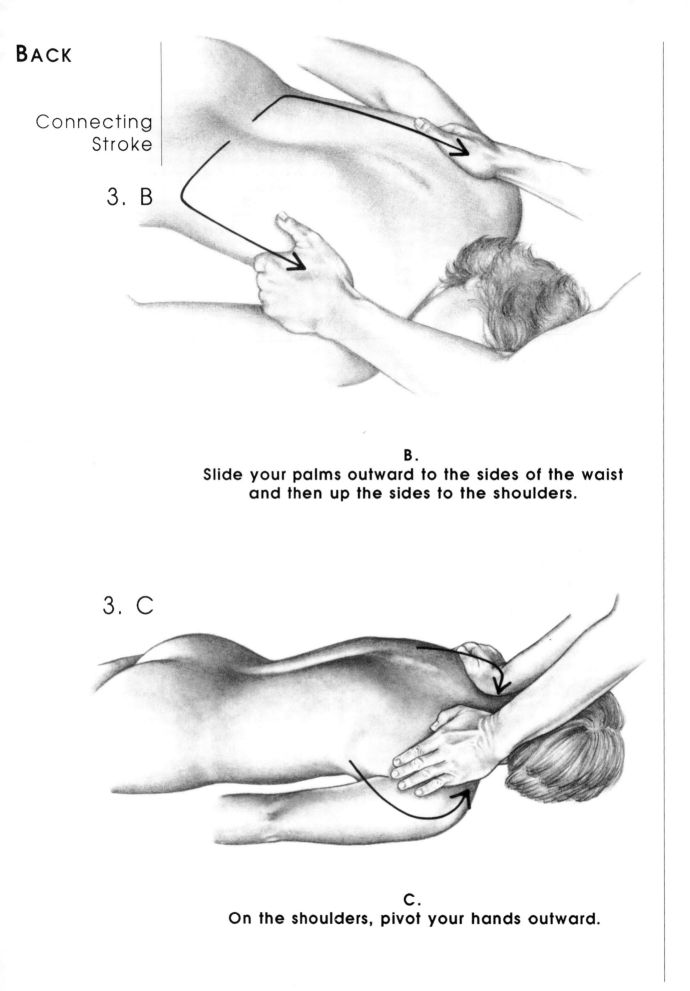

**B.**
**Slide your palms outward to the sides of the waist and then up the sides to the shoulders.**

3. C

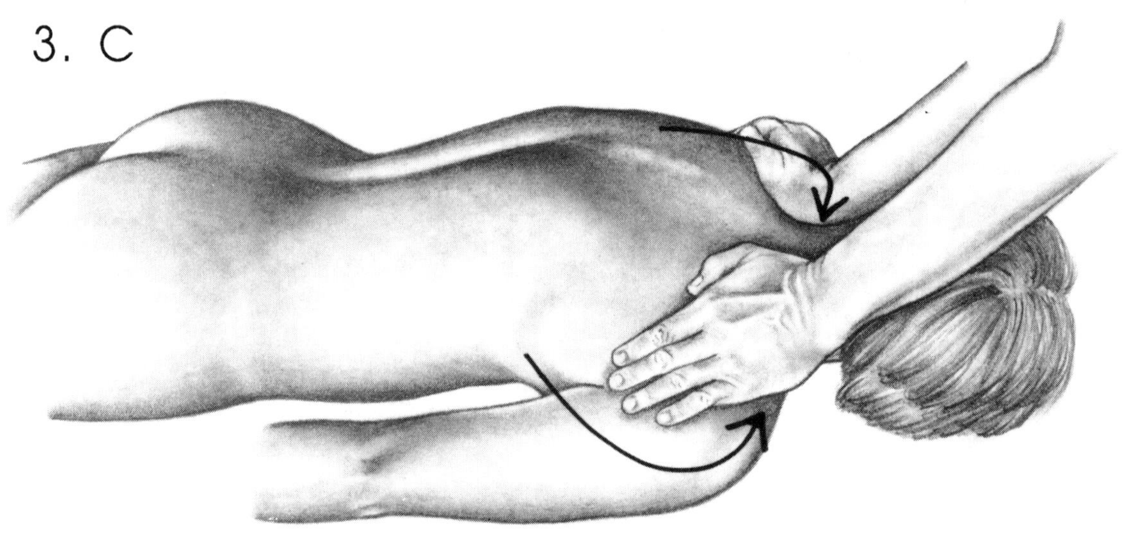

**C.**
**On the shoulders, pivot your hands outward.**

Connecting Stroke

3. D

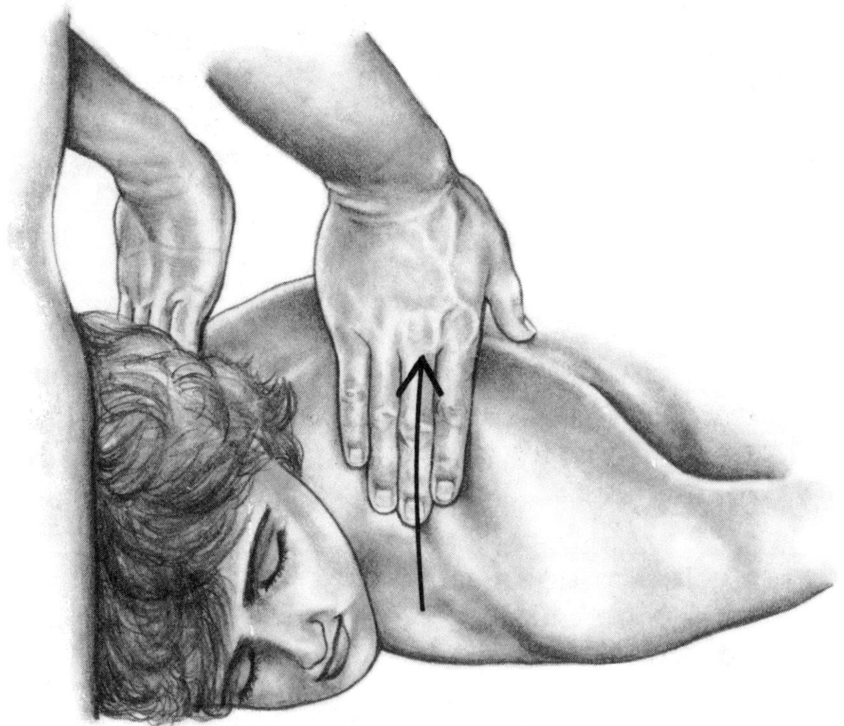

**D.**
**Slide upwards across the shoulder muscles (not the throat).**

**- - -**

**Repeat this whole stroke (A-D) several times.**

## 4. Prayer Stroke

Prayer Stroke

4. A

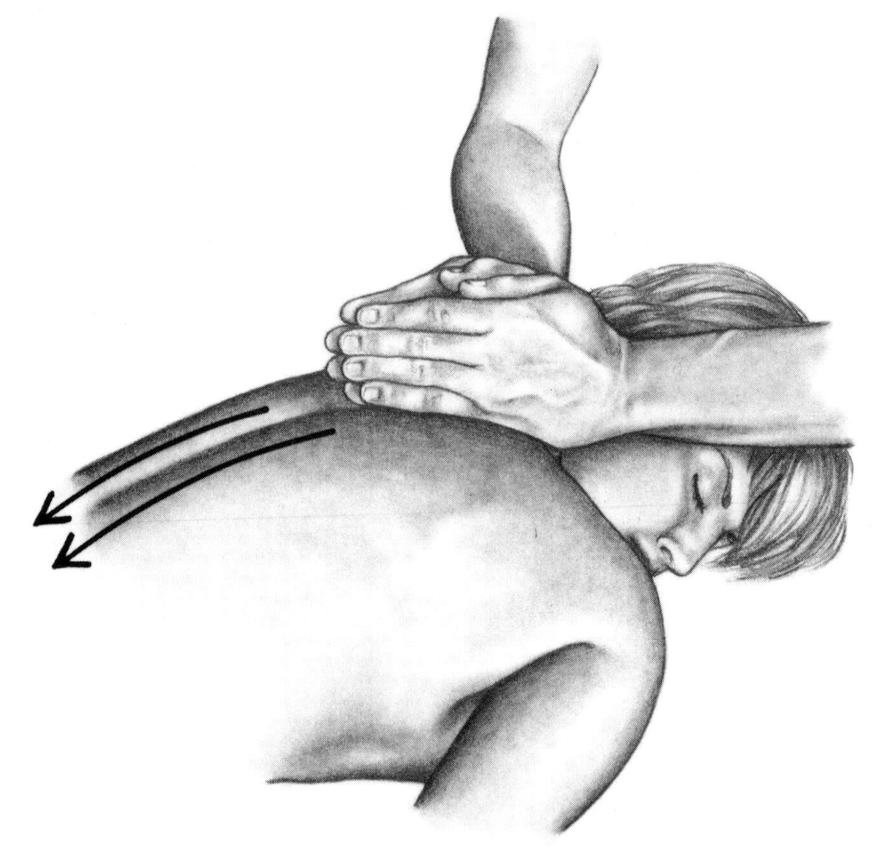

A.
Just to each side of the spine,
slide the outer edge of your hands
down the back to below the waist.

4. B

B.
(Now follow the same movements
as in the previous stroke, #3.)
Slide your palms outward to the sides of the waist
and then up the sides to the shoulders.

4. C

C.
On the shoulders, pivot your hands outward
(as in the previous stroke, #3).

4. D

D.
Slide upwards across the shoulder muscles
— not the throat
(as in the previous stroke, #3).

\- - -

Repeat this whole stroke (A-D) several times.

## 5. Shoulder Strokes

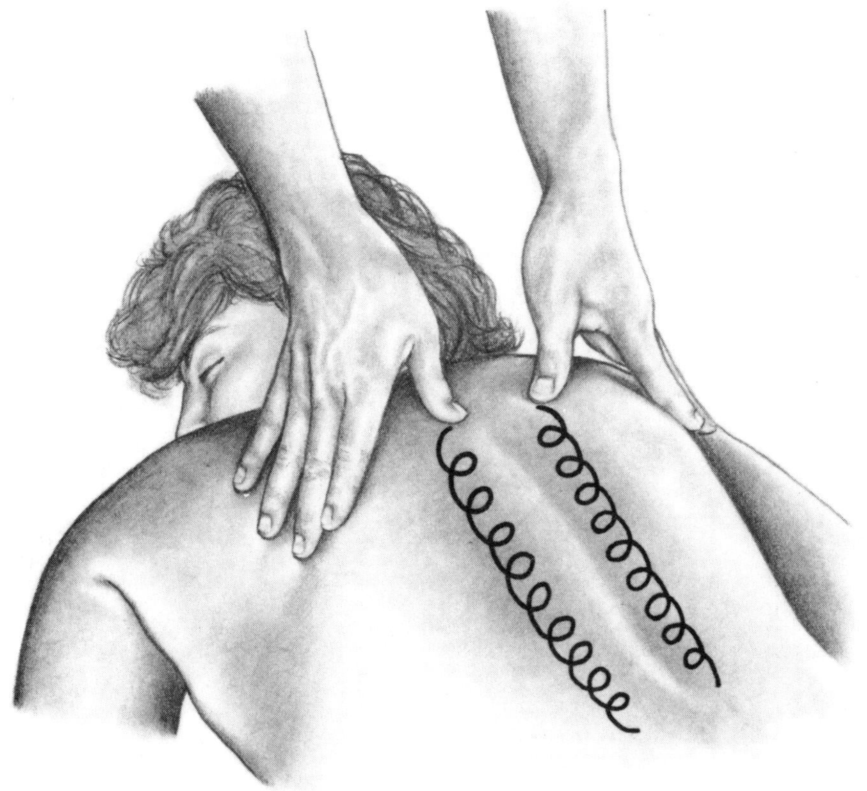

Shoulder Strokes

5. A

**A.**

**Just to each side of the spine,**
**make circles with the flat parts of your thumbs.**
**Here the thumbs mirror each other:**
**down together,**
**outward from spine together,**
**etc..**

**Focus the pressure**
**in the direction toward his/her feet.**
**Let your fingers remain in contact with your partner.**

**This series of circles gradually comes UP the back.**

Shoulder
Strokes

5. B

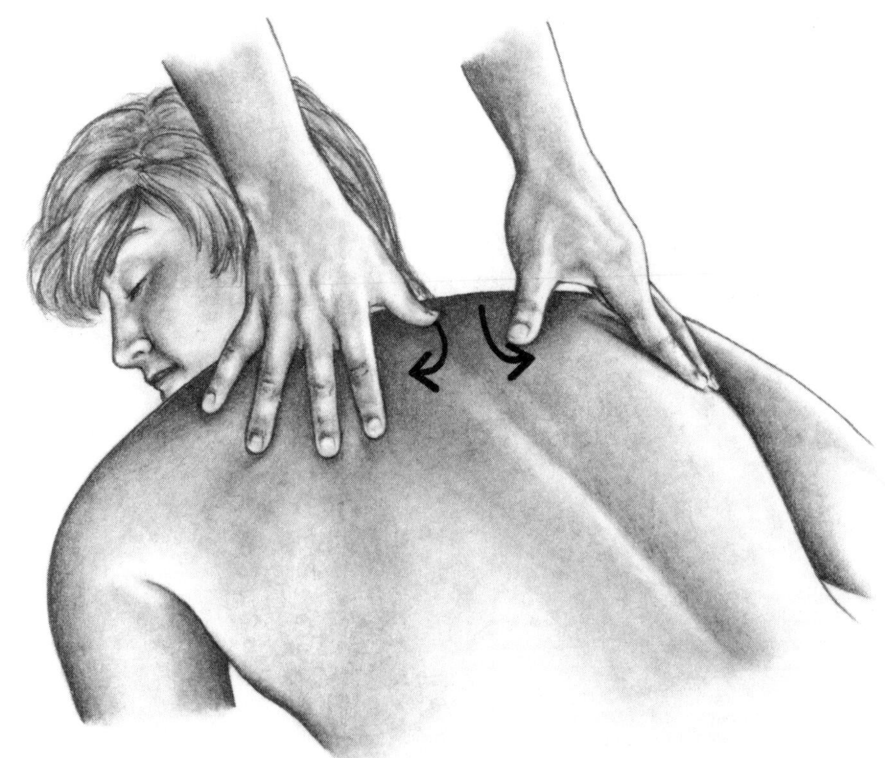

**B.**
**On the right shoulder between the spine and scapula, make circles with your thumbs — this time alternating your hands one after the other.**

**Focus on the area near the neck.**

Shoulder Strokes

5. C

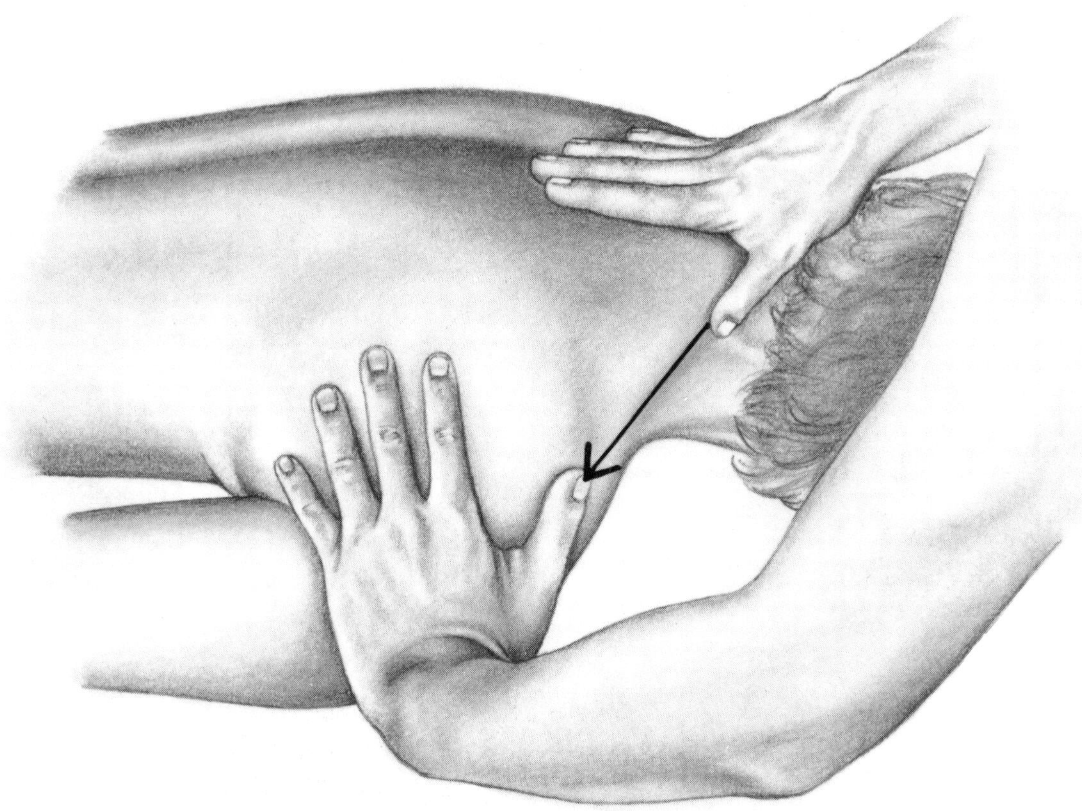

C.
On the groove between the right scapula and clavicle, slide your thumbs outward toward the shoulder tip — alternating one hand after the other.

5. D

D.
Now apply Parts B and C on the left shoulder.

## 6. Fingers' Pull

Fingers' Pull
6.

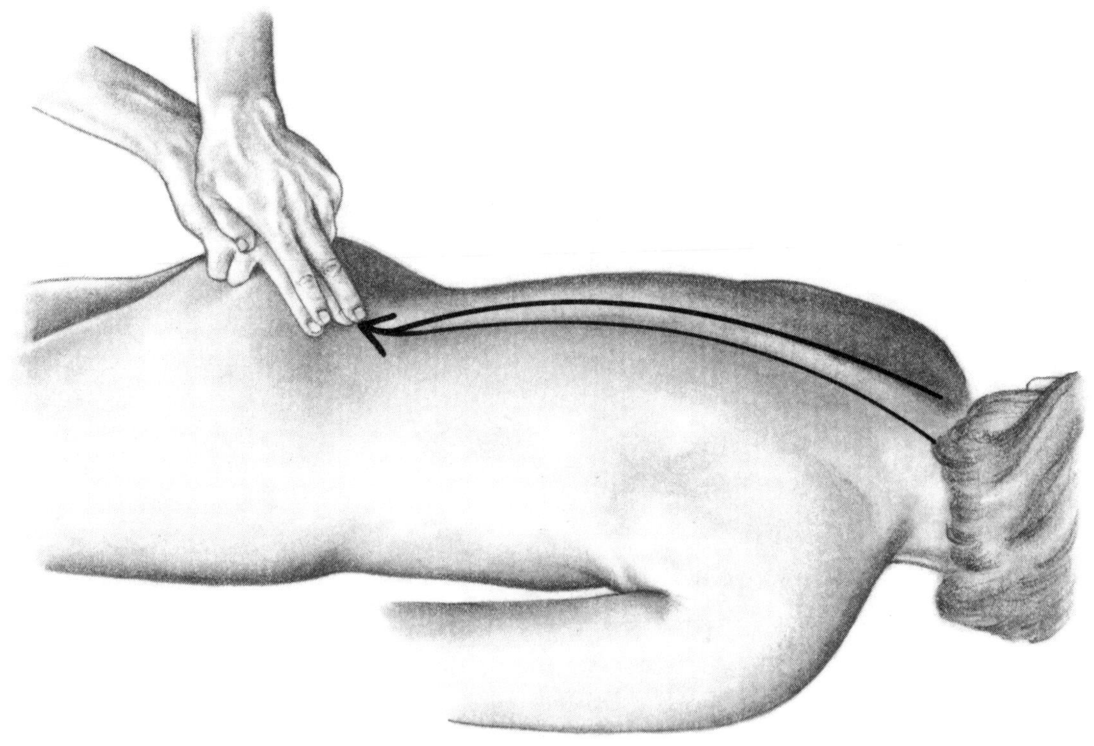

With a finger pad
on each side of the spine at the neck,
pull downward toward the buttocks.
Use a firm pressure.
(You can have even more pressure
by putting the fingers of your other hand
on top of the first.)

- - -

Repeat this whole stroke several times.

## 7. Side Pulling

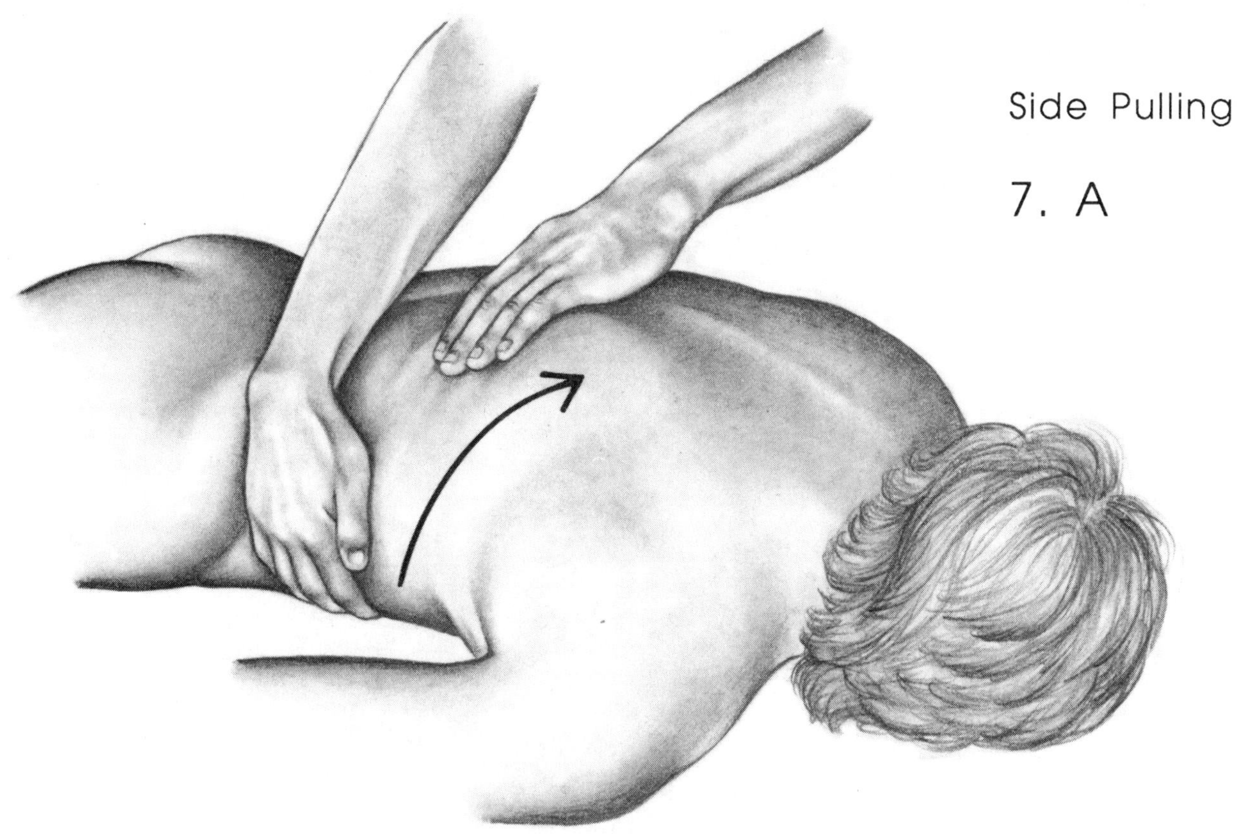

Side Pulling

7. A

**A.**
**Alternating your hands on one side, slide them in a pulling manner across the side of the torso toward the spine.**

**(This series includes the area from the hips to near the underarms.)**

7. B

**B.**
**Move to the other side, and apply the pulling movements to the opposite side.**

# BACK OF LEGS

Instructions: Written as applied to the right leg.
Your Position: Initially, to the right of the right foot.

## 8. Connecting Stroke

Connecting Stroke

8. A

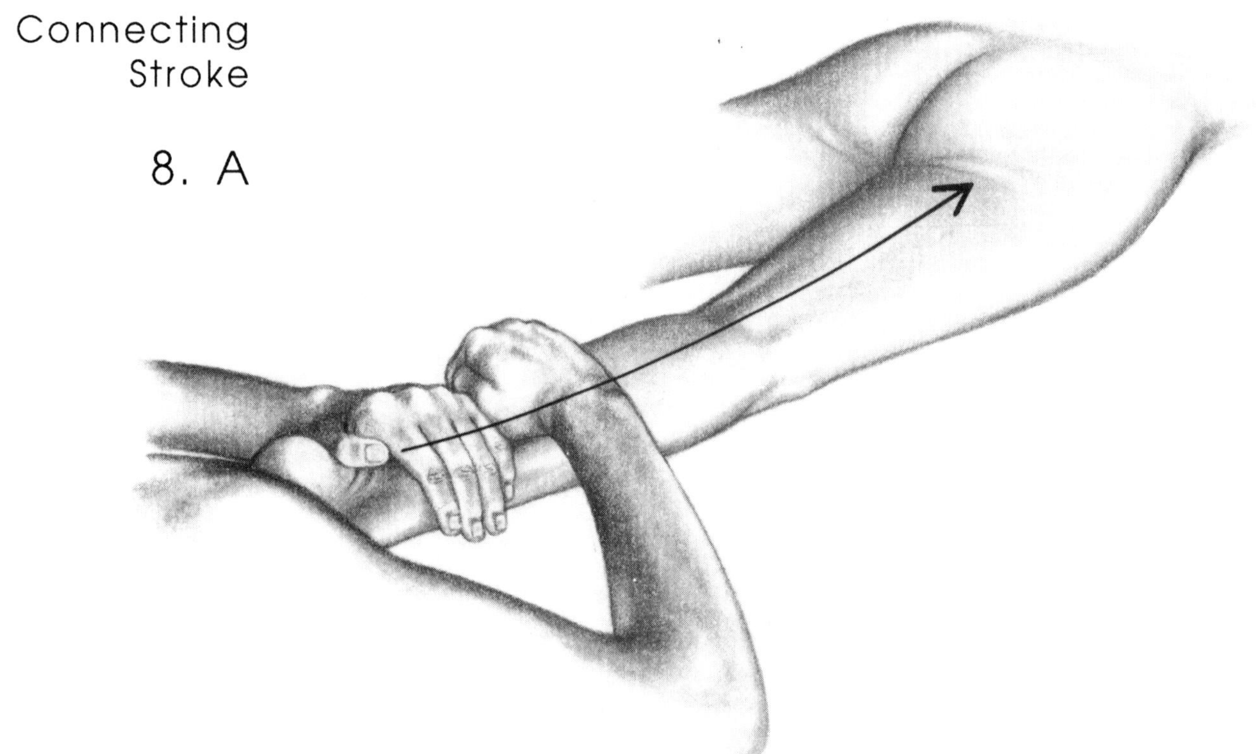

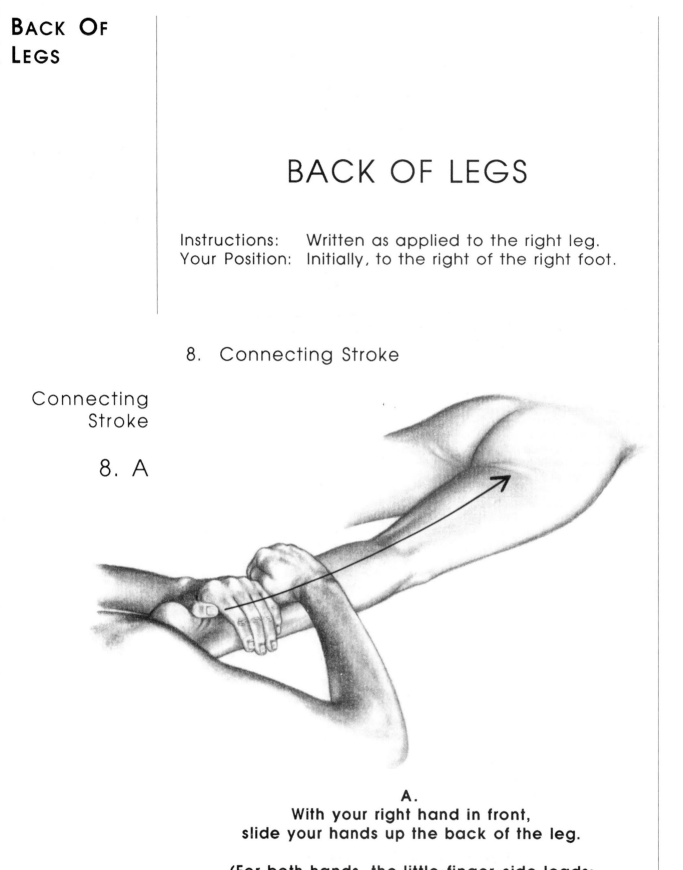

**A.**
**With your right hand in front, slide your hands up the back of the leg.**

**(For both hands, the little-finger-side leads; the thumbs are beside their index fingers.)**

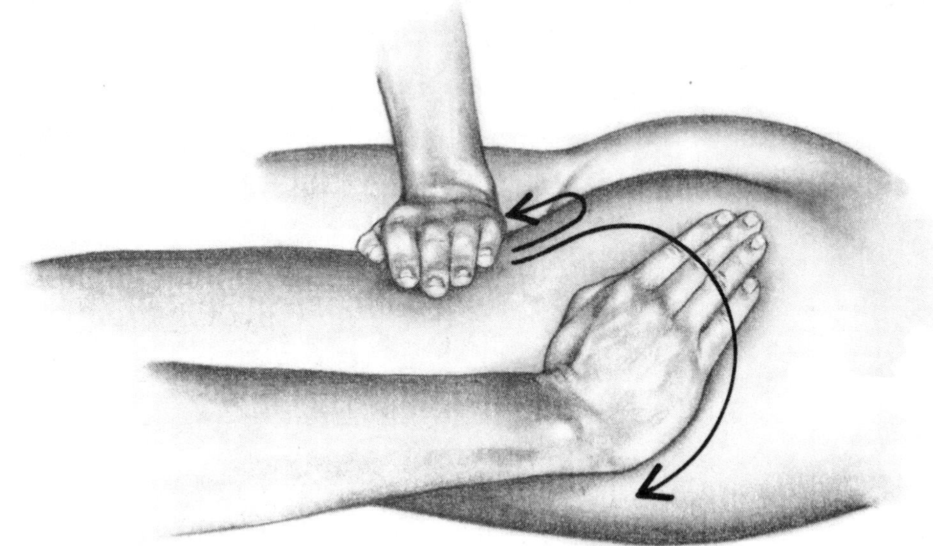

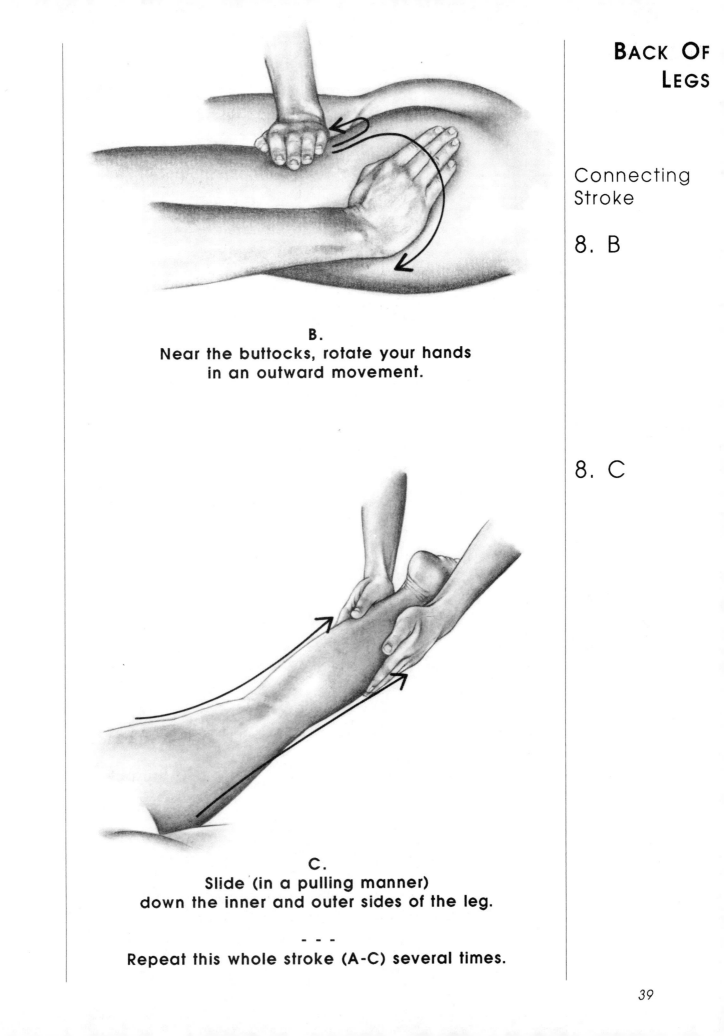

Connecting Stroke

8. B

**B.**
**Near the buttocks, rotate your hands in an outward movement.**

8. C

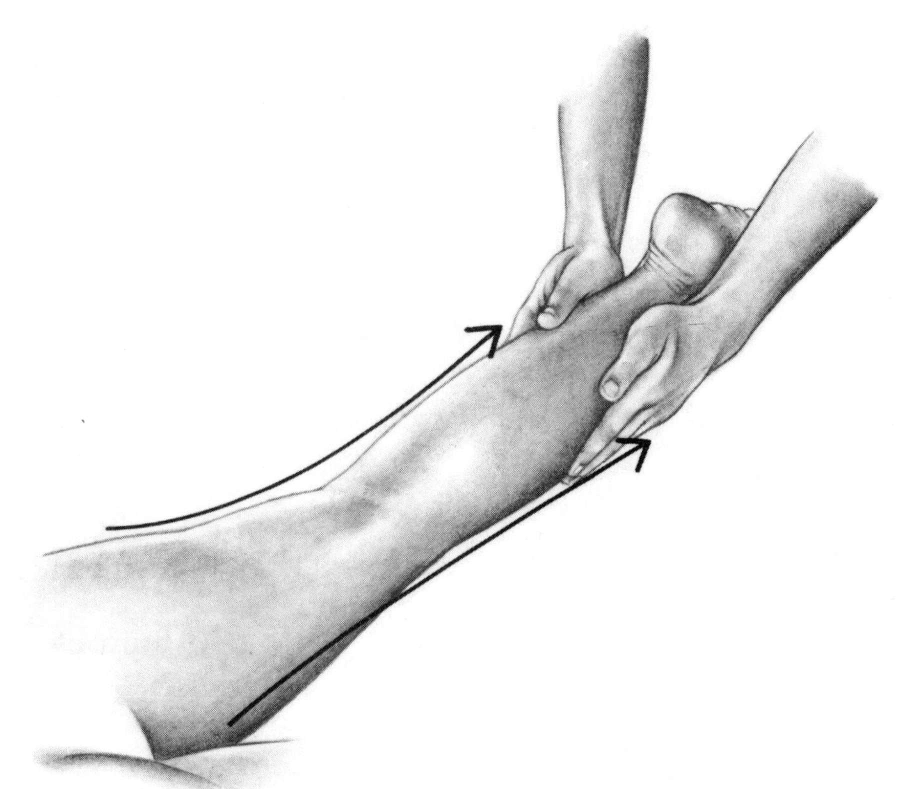

**C.**
**Slide (in a pulling manner) down the inner and outer sides of the leg.**

**- - -**

**Repeat this whole stroke (A-C) several times.**

Kneading

9.

## 9. Kneading

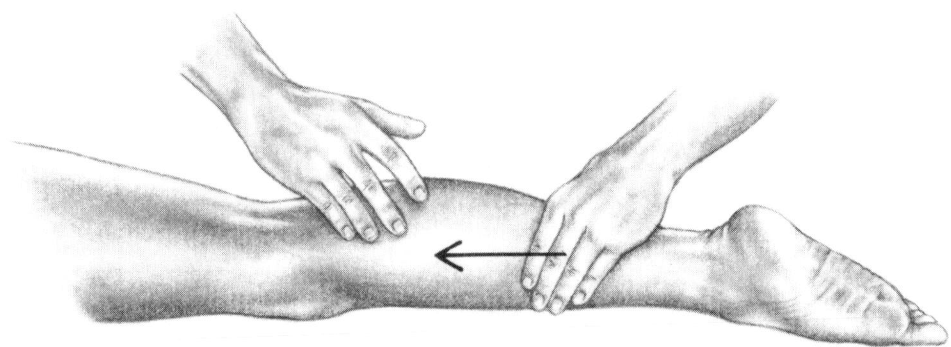

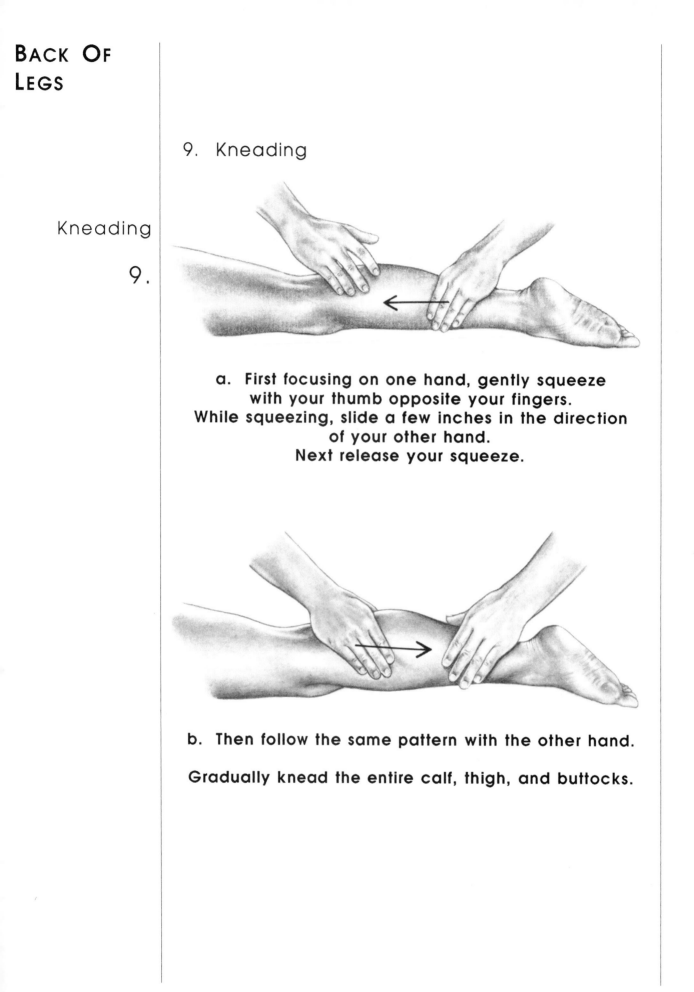

**a. First focusing on one hand, gently squeeze with your thumb opposite your fingers. While squeezing, slide a few inches in the direction of your other hand. Next release your squeeze.**

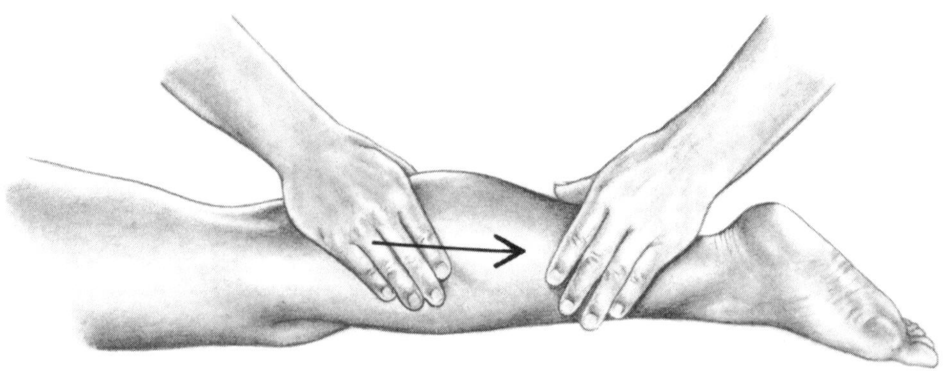

**b. Then follow the same pattern with the other hand.**

**Gradually knead the entire calf, thigh, and buttocks.**

10. Thumb Slide

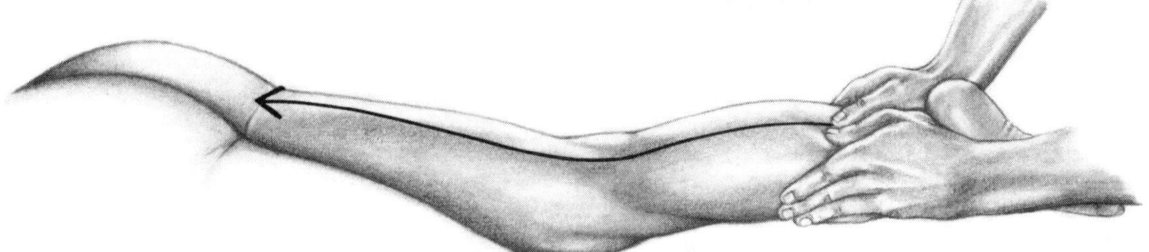

Thumb Slide

10. A

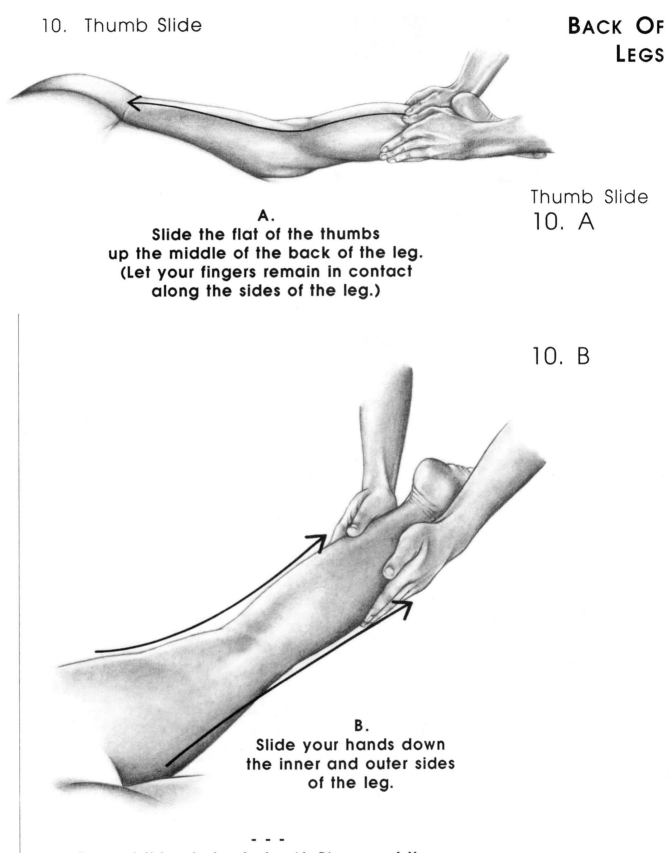

**A.**
**Slide the flat of the thumbs up the middle of the back of the leg. (Let your fingers remain in contact along the sides of the leg.)**

10. B

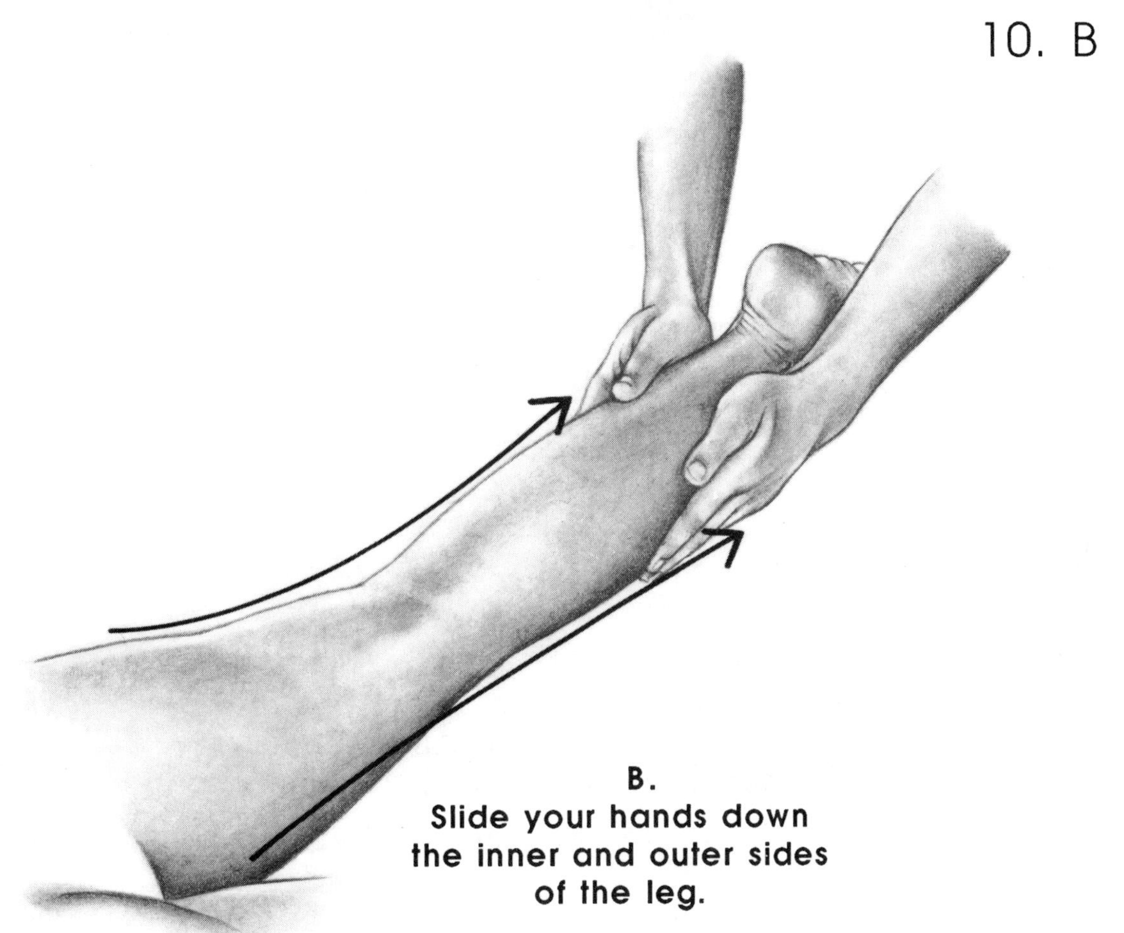

**B.**
**Slide your hands down the inner and outer sides of the leg.**

\- - -

**Repeat this whole stroke (A-B) several times.**

V Stroke

11. A

## 11. V Stroke

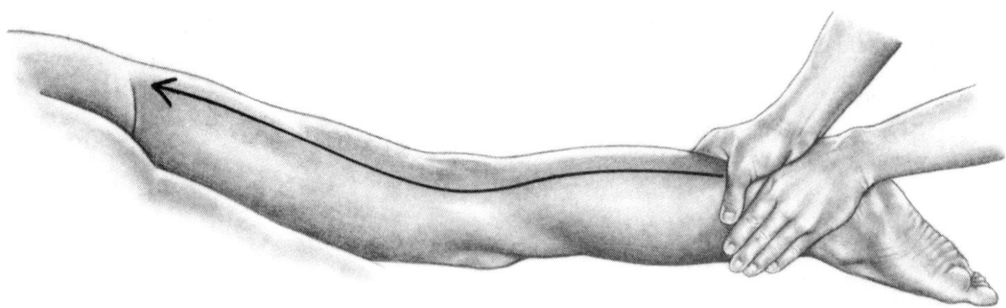

**A.**
**Slide your hands in a V shape up the back of the leg. To form a "V," form both hands as if to shake hands. Then place the right hand above the left hand so that the right little finger is on the left thumb and the right thumb is on the left index finger.**

11. B

**B.**
**Slide down the inner and outer sides of the leg (as in the previous stroke, #10).**

\- - -

**Repeat this whole stroke (A-B) several times.**

Repeat #8
12.

## 12. Repeat:

Back-Of-Leg Connecting Stroke (#8).

Feather Stroke
13.

## 13. Back-Of-Leg Feather Stroke

**Alternating your hands in a pulling movement, delicately stroke your fingertips over the entire leg — sometimes short strokes, sometimes long ones.**

Same Sequence on Left Leg
14.

## 14. Follow the same sequence on the left leg.

**Remember to reverse your right- and left-hand positions.**

# BACK SIDE CONCLUSION

Back Hug

15. Back Hug

15. A

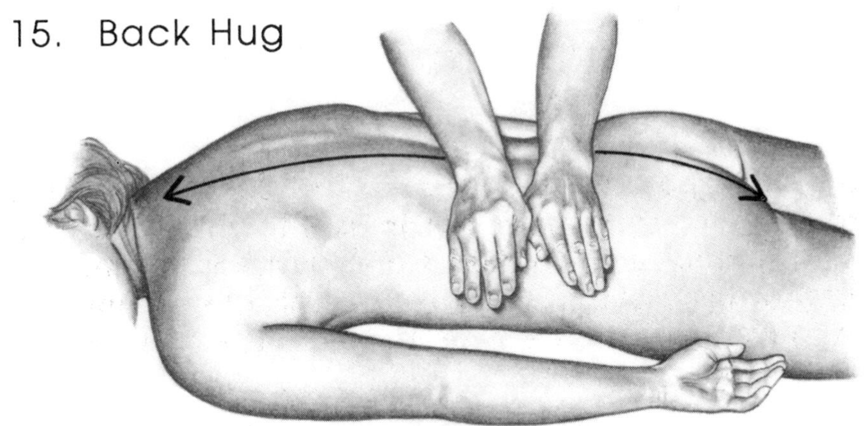

A.

(This may be a difficult stroke unless you are using a massage table.)

Using the soft, inner side of your forearms, begin at your lover's lower back and slide them to below the buttocks and to the upper back.

Then slide your forearms back together.

Repeat this whole movement several times.

15. B

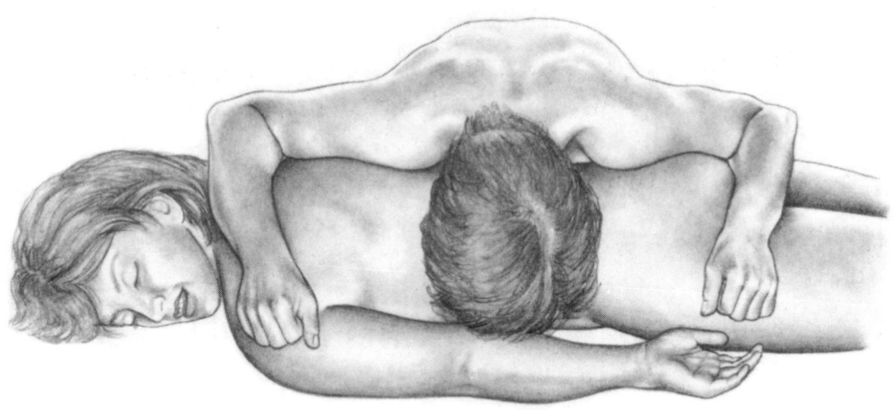

B.

After a few repetitions of Part A, rest your chest on the back.

Be very careful not to put pressure on the neck and throat area.

Concluding Stroke

16.

## 16. Concluding Stroke

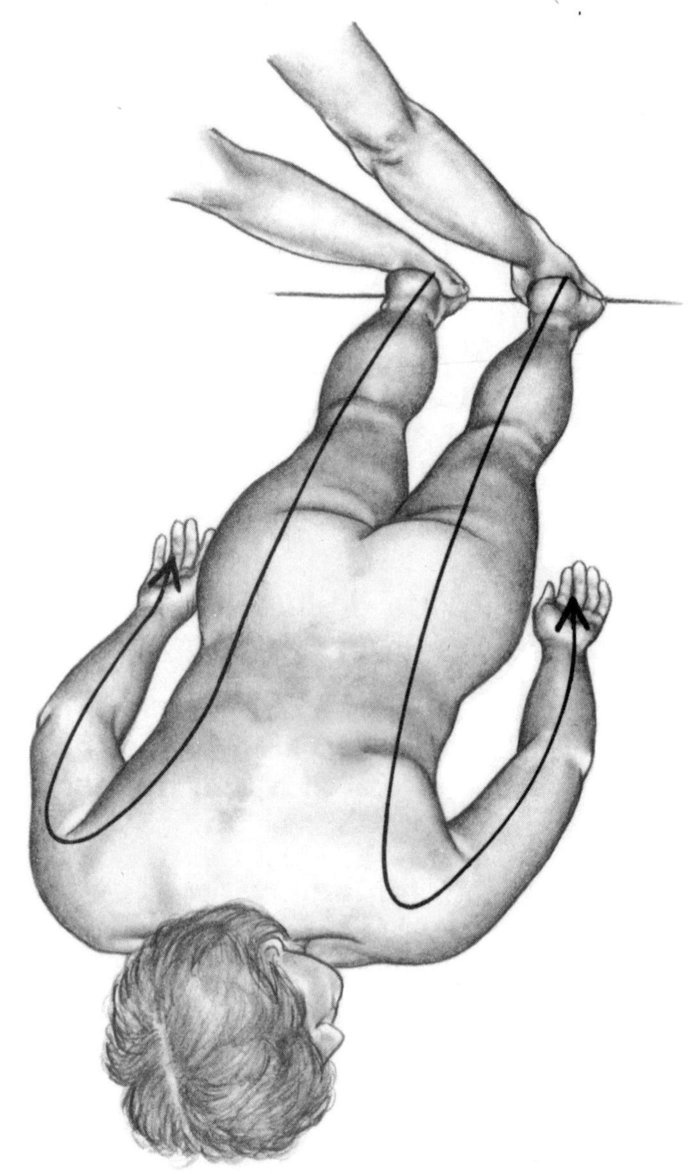

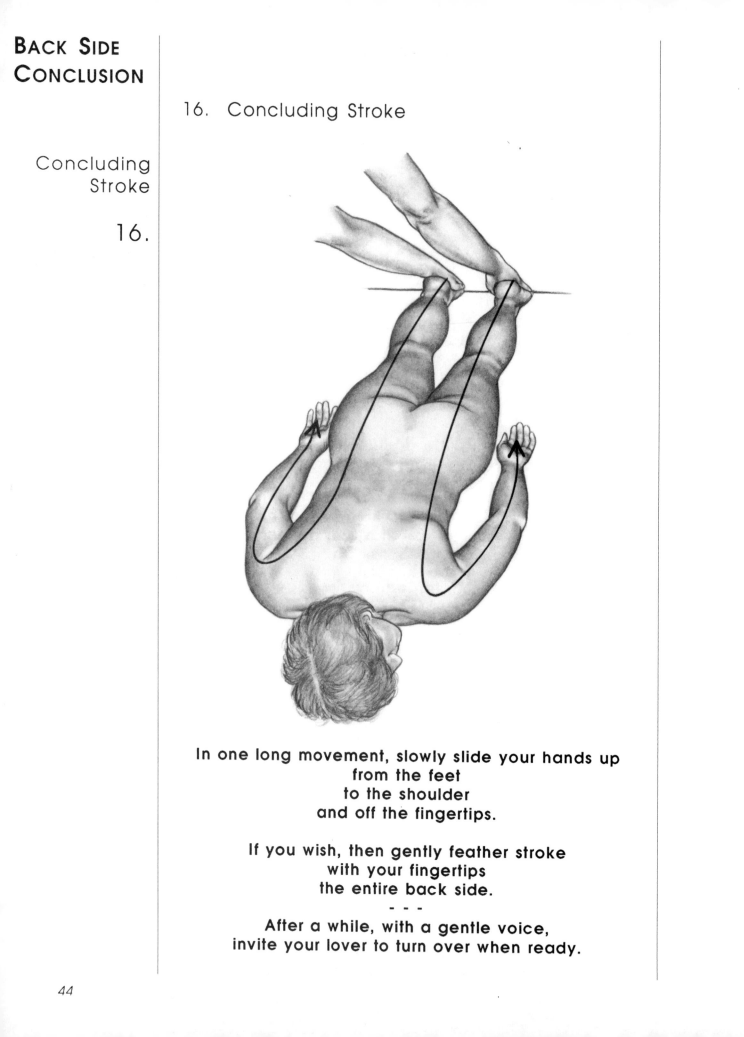

**In one long movement, slowly slide your hands up**
**from the feet**
**to the shoulder**
**and off the fingertips.**

**If you wish, then gently feather stroke**
**with your fingertips**
**the entire back side.**

**- - -**

**After a while, with a gentle voice,**
**invite your lover to turn over when ready.**

# ARMS



Instructions: Written as applied to the right arm.
Lover's Position: Lying on back with arms by side.
Your Position: Initially at the right waist, facing the head.

## 17. Connecting Stroke

Connecting Stroke

17. A

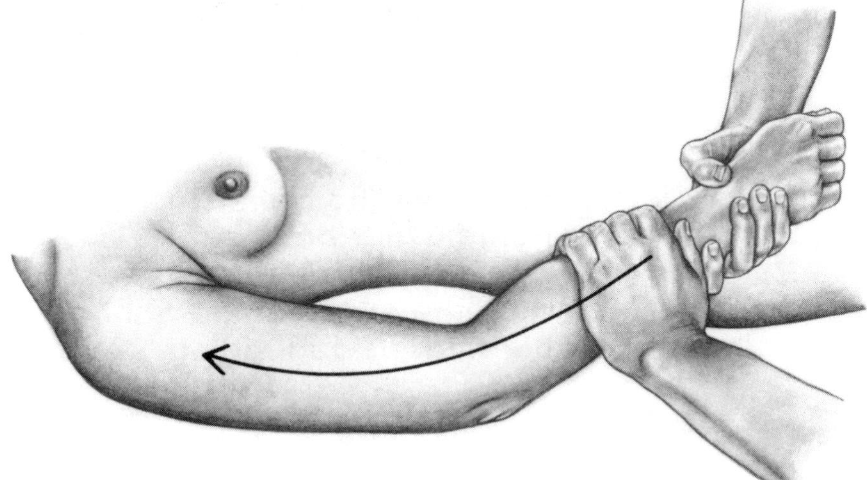

**A.**
**First, gently hold the right wrist in your right hand. Then with the little-finger side leading, slide your left hand up the outside of the right arm.**

17. B

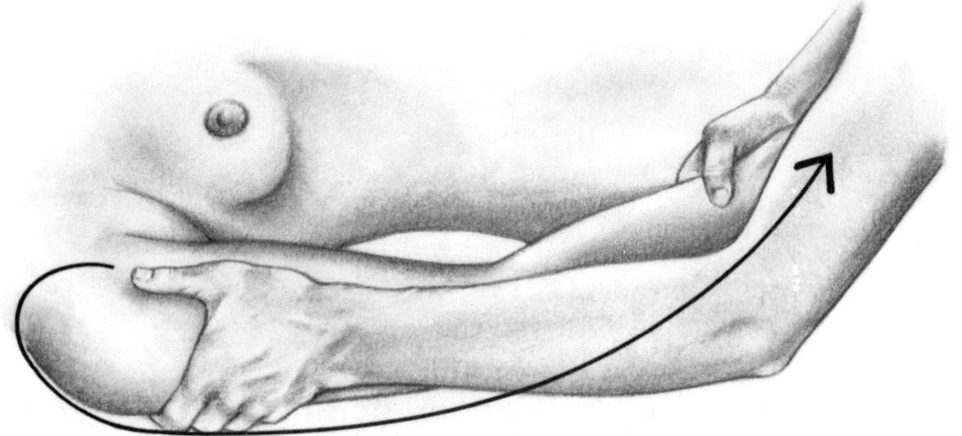

**B.**
**Pivot on the shoulder tip and slide down on the back side of the arm.**

Connecting Stroke

17. C

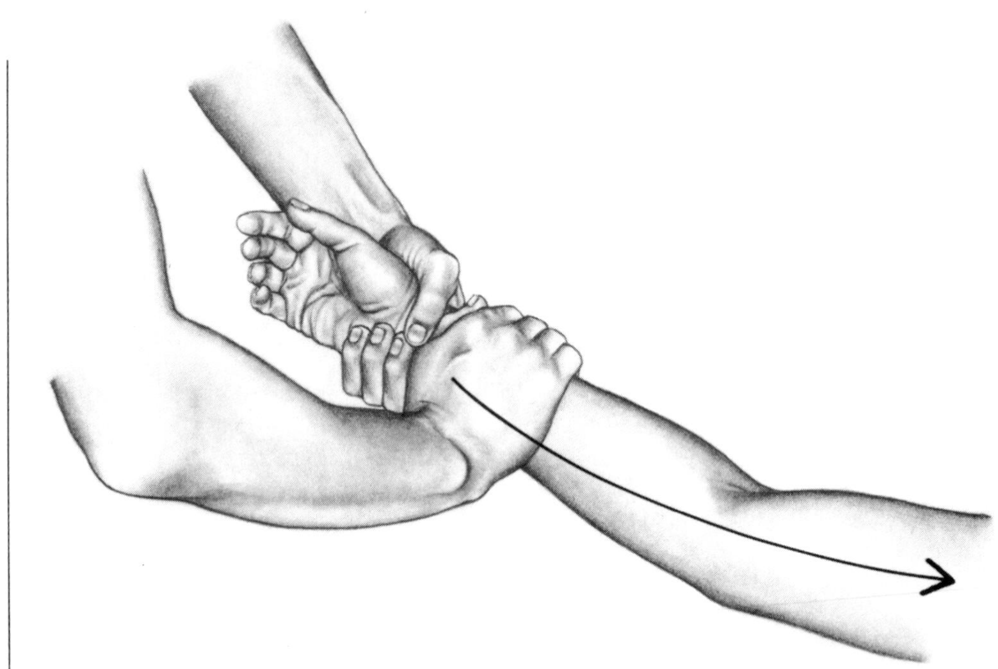

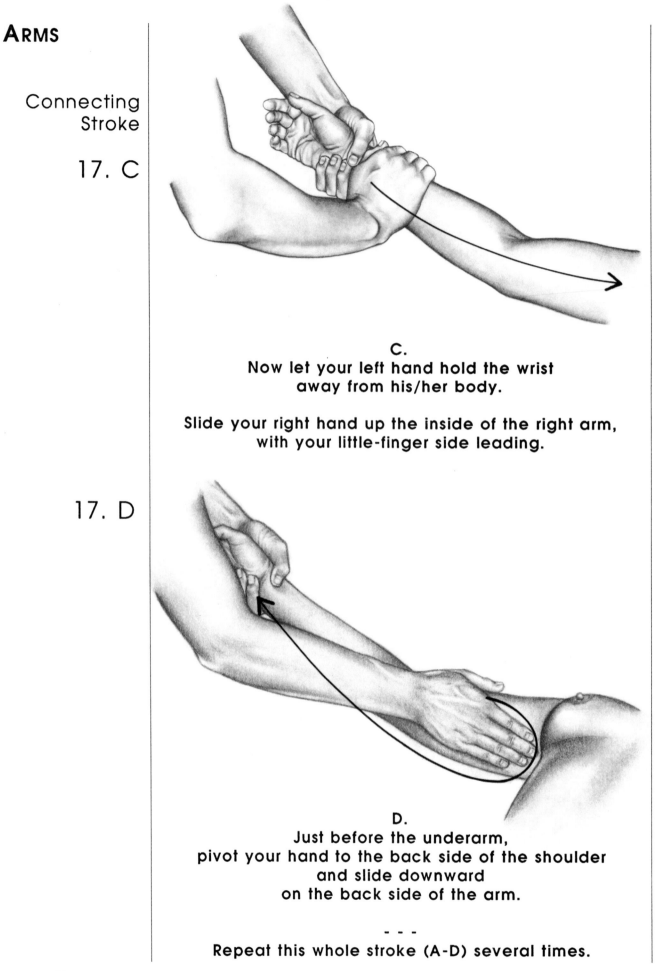

C.
Now let your left hand hold the wrist away from his/her body.

Slide your right hand up the inside of the right arm, with your little-finger side leading.

17. D

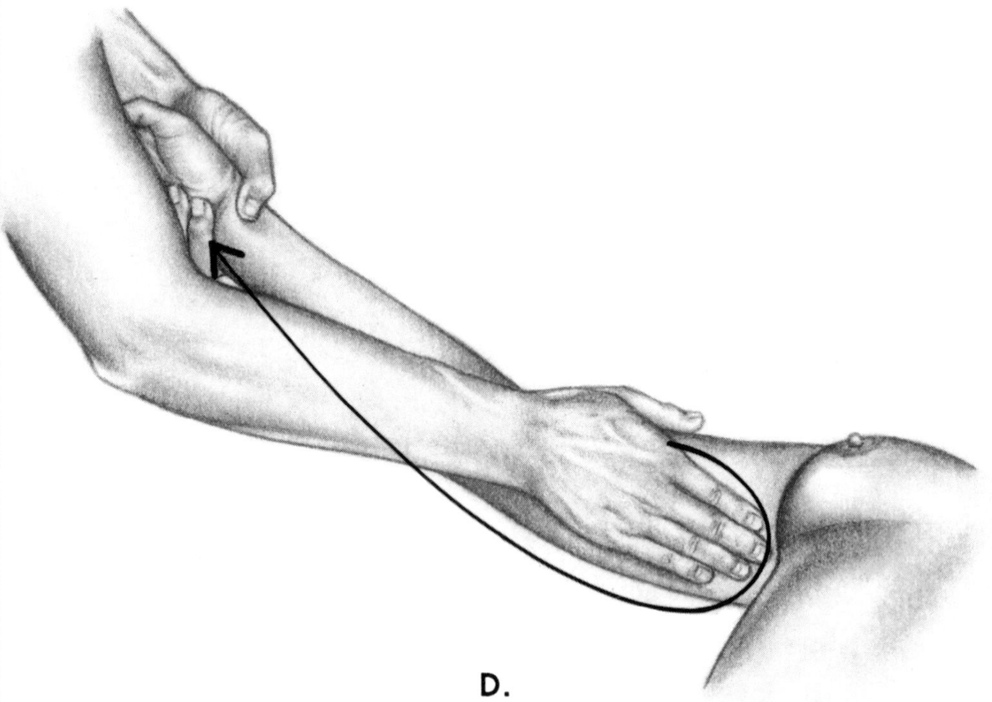

D.
Just before the underarm, pivot your hand to the back side of the shoulder and slide downward on the back side of the arm.

- - -

Repeat this whole stroke (A-D) several times.

## 18. Upper Arm Stroke

Upper Arm Stroke

18. A

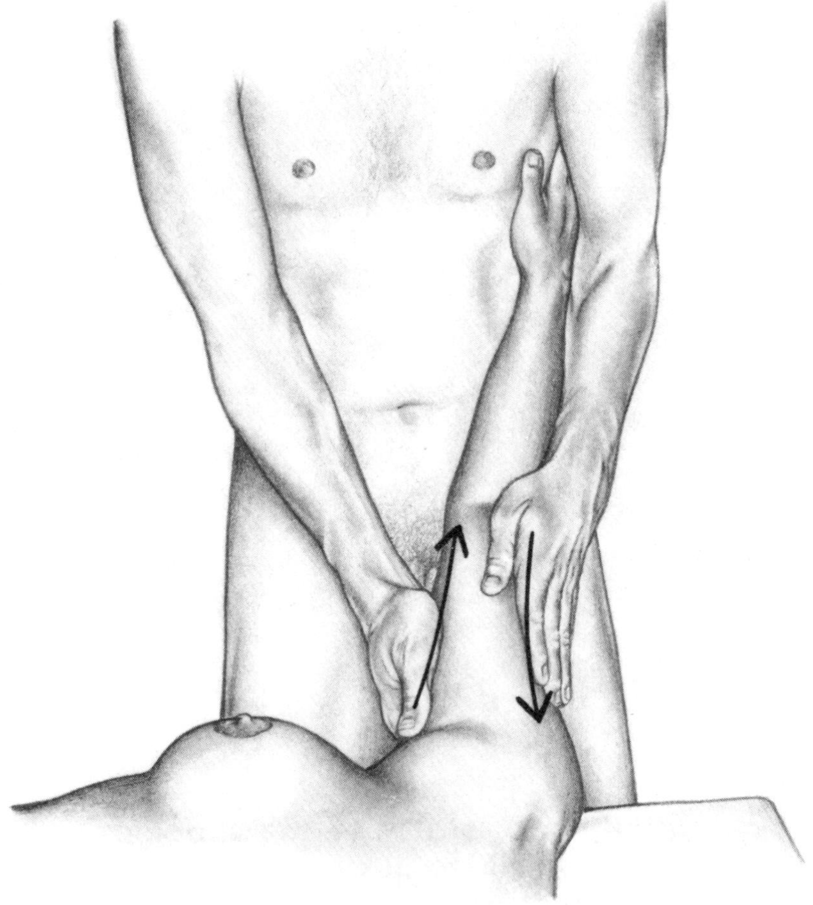

**A.**
**Hold the right hand on your left rib cage.**

**Slide your left hand upward on the outside of his/her upper arm**

**while your right hand slides downward on the back side.**

Upper Arm Stroke

18. B

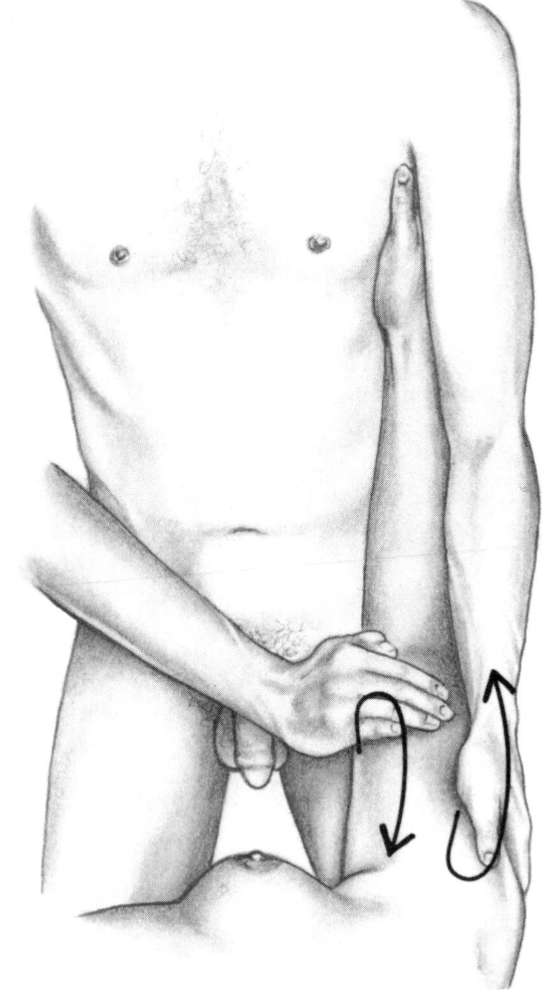

**B.**

**Your left hand rotates on the shoulder**
**and slides downward**
**on the back side of the upper arm**

**while your right hand rotates at the elbow**
**and slides upward**
**on the upper side of the upper arm.**

18. C

**C.**

**Your left hand rotates at the elbow**
**and slides upward**
**on the outside of the upper arm**
**(which is Part A again)**

**while your right hand rotates at the underarm**
**and slides downward**
**on the back side**
**(which is Part A again).**

**- - -**

**Repeat this whole stroke (A-C) several times.**

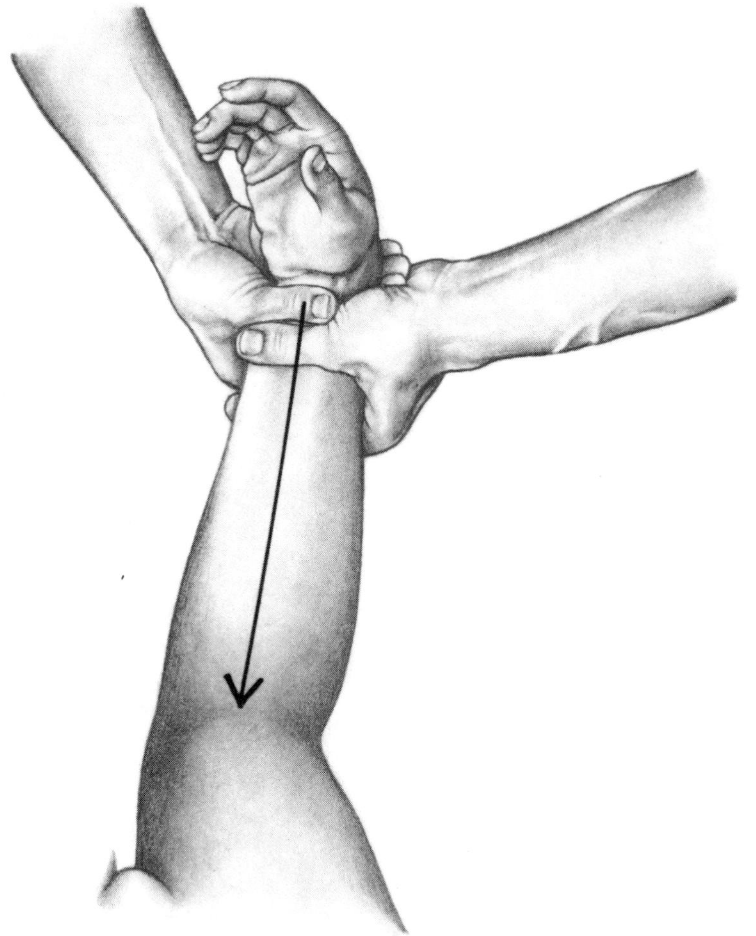

Forearm Stroke

19. A

19. Forearm Stroke

**A.**

**Holding the forearm upright,
slide the flat sides of your thumbs
down the inside of the forearm.
Let your thumbs be parallel with each other.**

19. B

**B.**

**When your thumbs reach the inner side of the elbow,
lighten your touch
and slide your hands back up to the wrist.**

**- - -**

**Continue with the right hand
before massaging the left arm.**

# HANDS

Instructions: Written as applied to the right hand.

## 20. Hand Curl

Hand Curl

20.

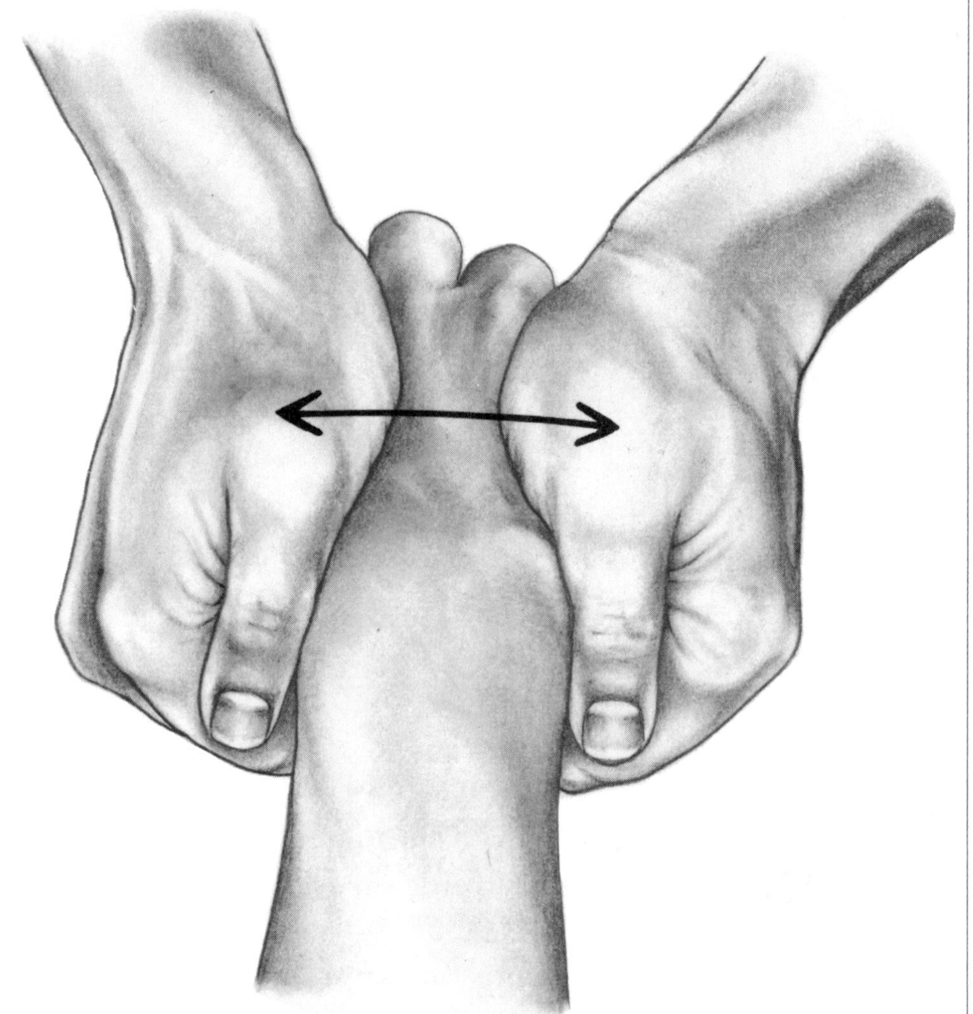

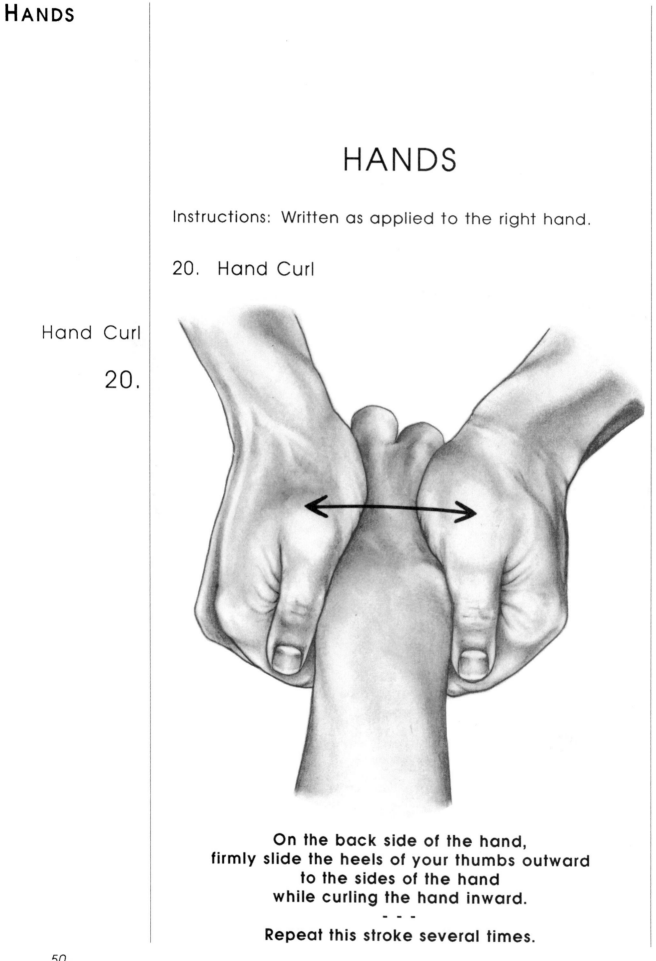

**On the back side of the hand,
firmly slide the heels of your thumbs outward
to the sides of the hand
while curling the hand inward.**

**- - -**

**Repeat this stroke several times.**

## 21. Palm Massage

Palm Massage

21.

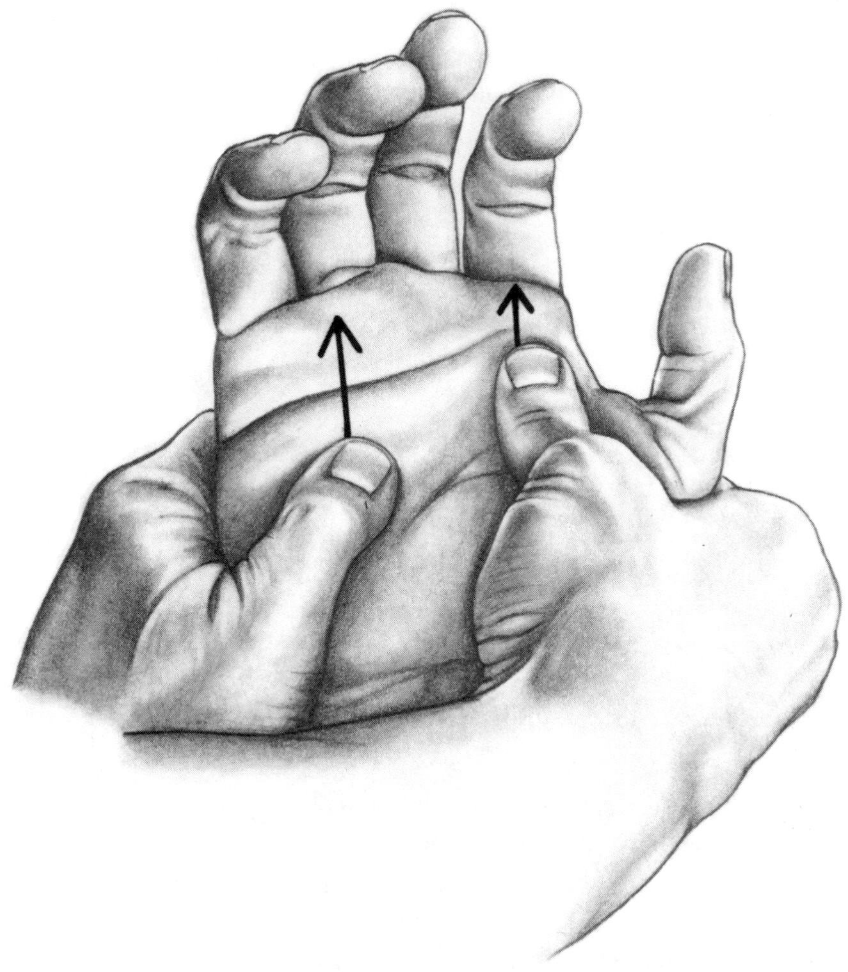

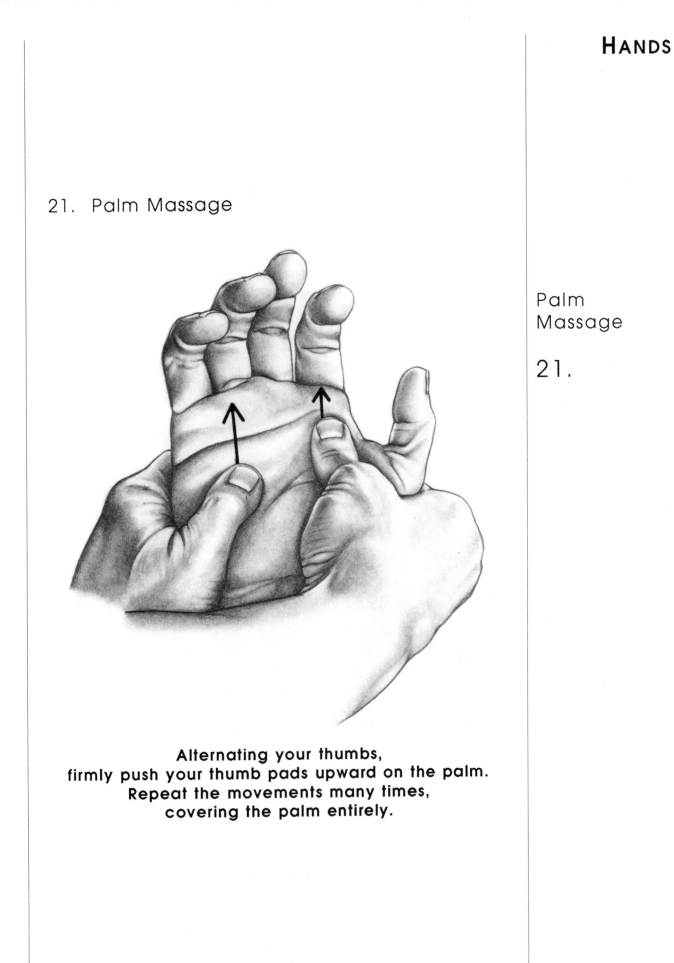

**Alternating your thumbs, firmly push your thumb pads upward on the palm. Repeat the movements many times, covering the palm entirely.**

Web Stroke

22.

22. Web Stroke

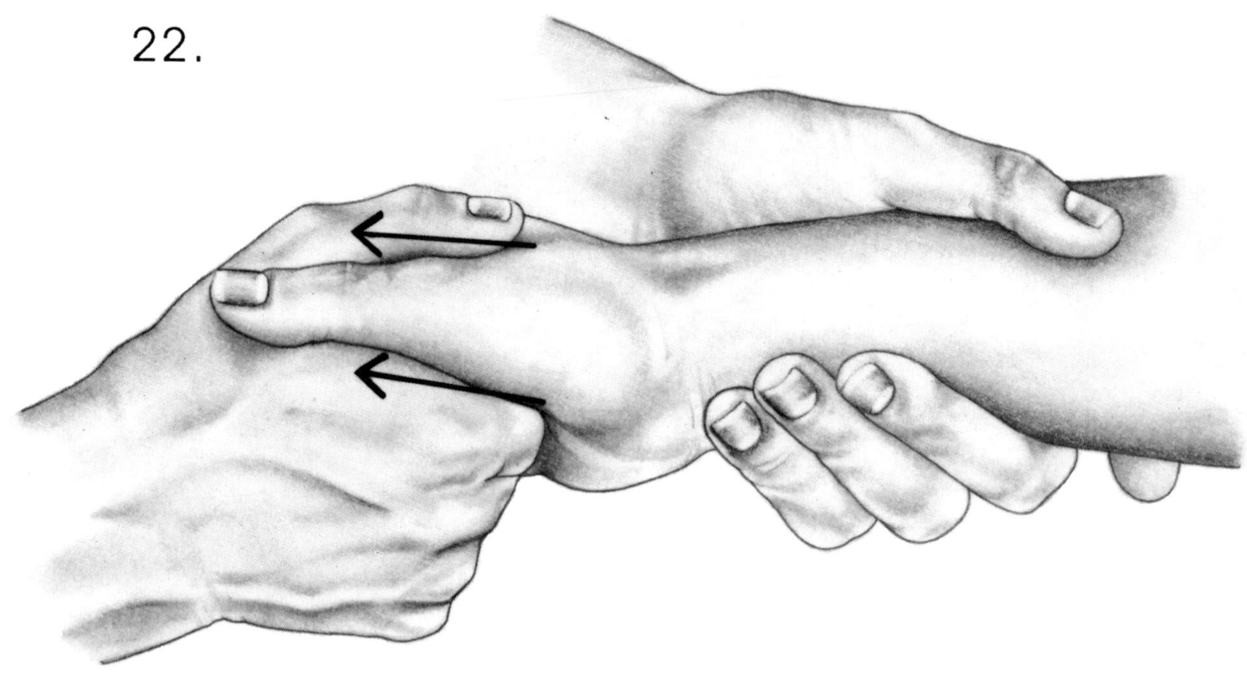

**With your right thumb and curled index finger between the right thumb and first finger, slide outward firmly.**

**- - -**

**Repeat this stroke several times.**

## 23. Finger Stroke

Finger Stroke

23. A

**A.**
**Starting at the tip of the finger, slide very lightly down the sides of the finger with your thumb and finger — very, very lightly.**

23. B

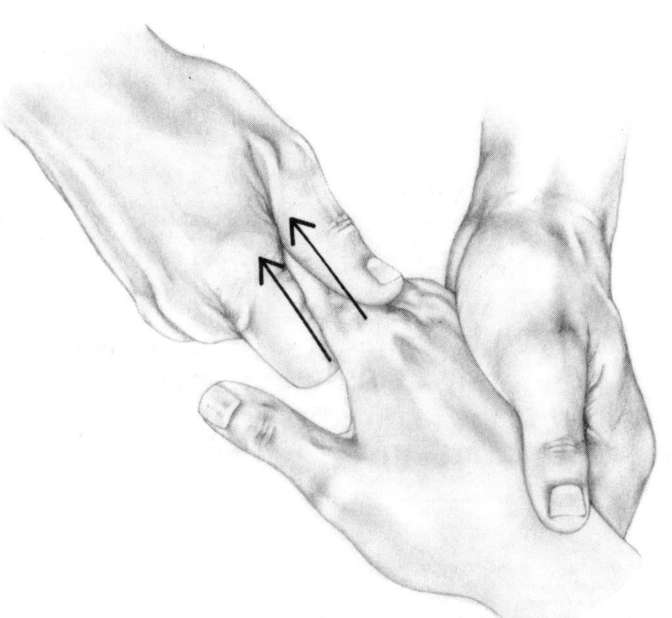

**B.**
**Grasping the finger firmly at its base, slide up and off the finger.**

**- - -**

**Repeat Part A and Part B once on the thumb and once on each finger.**

Palm Reading

24.

## 24. Palm Reading

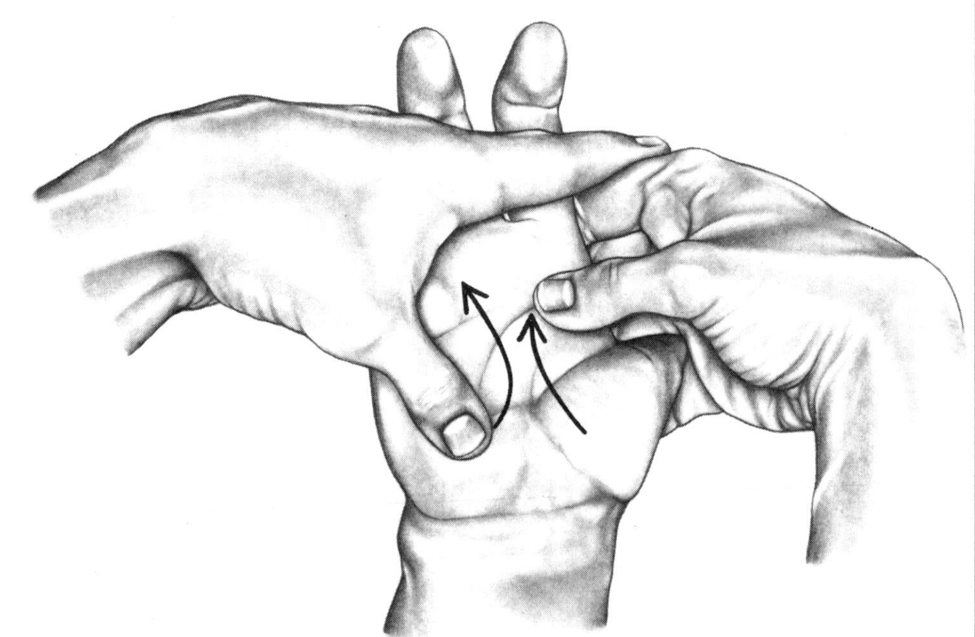

**Interlacing your fingers with your lover's, stretch the palm open and lightly feather stroke the palm with your thumb tips — very, very, very lightly.**

Repeat #17

25.

## 25. Repeat: Arm Connecting Stroke (#17)

Feather Stroke

26.

## 26. Arm and Hand Feather Stroke

**Alternating your hands in a pulling movement, delicately stroke your fingertips over the entire arm and hand — sometimes short strokes, sometimes long ones.**

Same Arm and Hand Sequence on Left Arm

27.

## 27. Follow the same Arm and Hand sequence on the left arm.

**Remember to reverse your right- and left-hand positions.**

# FRONT OF LEGS

Instructions: Written as applied to the right leg.

## 28. Connecting Stroke

28. A

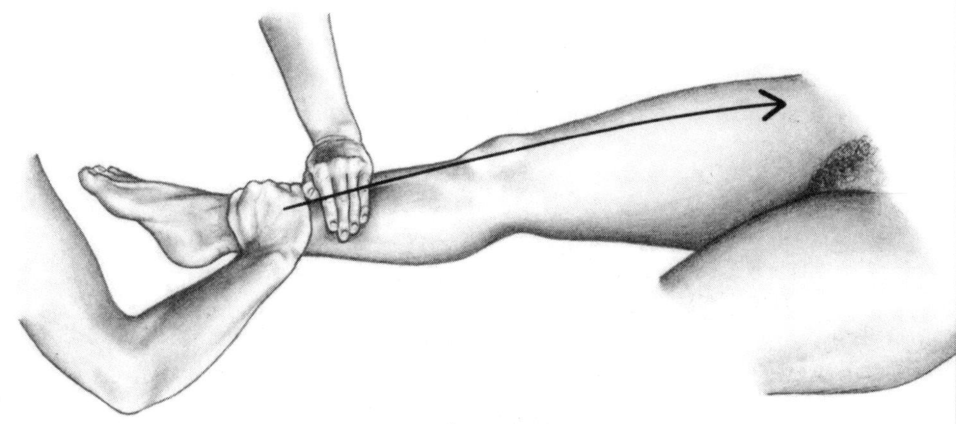

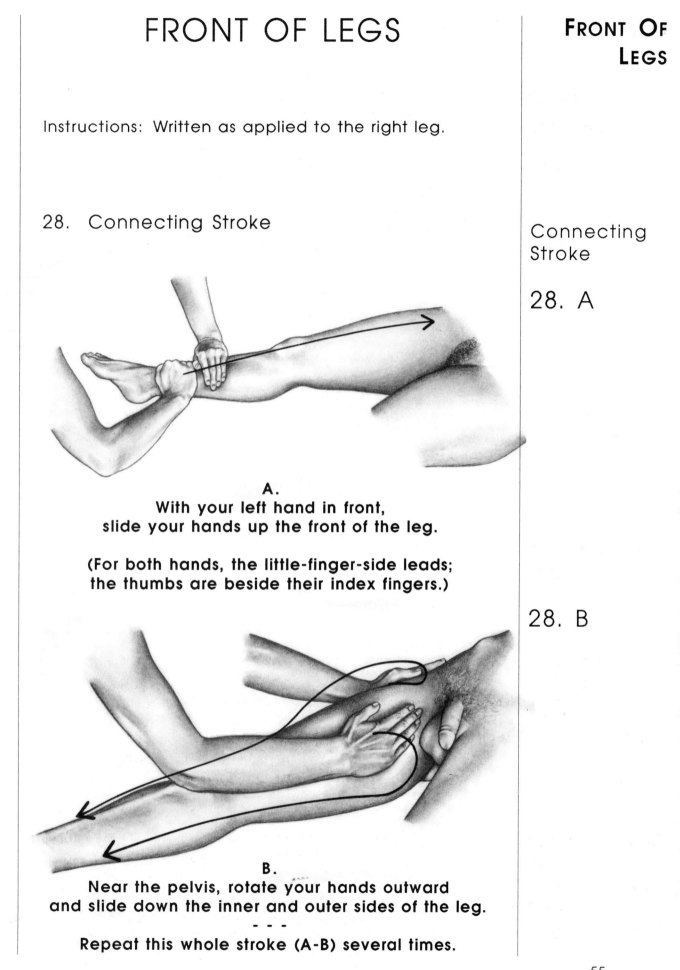

**A.**
**With your left hand in front,**
**slide your hands up the front of the leg.**

**(For both hands, the little-finger-side leads;**
**the thumbs are beside their index fingers.)**

28. B

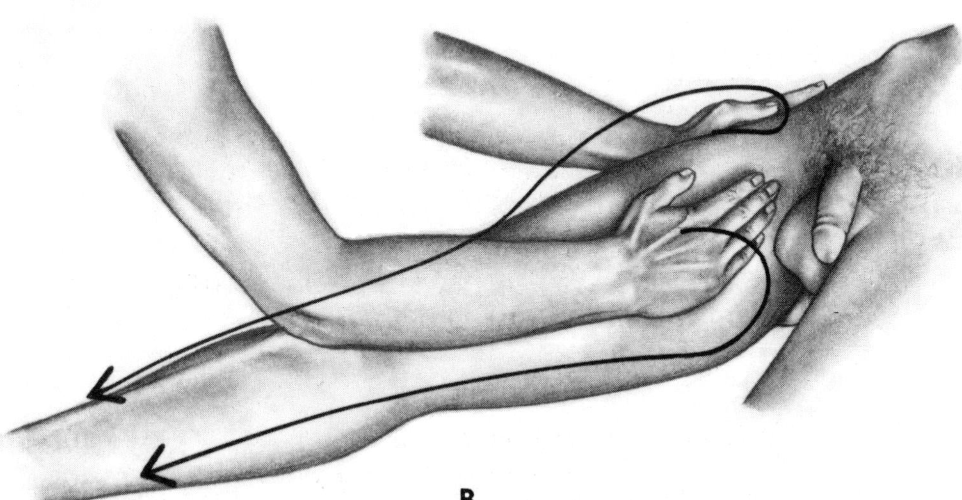

**B.**
**Near the pelvis, rotate your hands outward**
**and slide down the inner and outer sides of the leg.**

**- - -**

**Repeat this whole stroke (A-B) several times.**

Mini-Connecting Stroke

29.

## 29. Mini-Connecting Stroke

**On the thigh,
make a series of connecting strokes
similar to the previous stroke (#28)
but shorter and only on the thigh.**

**Each succeeding stroke starts
a little farther up the thigh
and ends a little farther up.**

**Repeat this whole series several times.**

Thigh Kneading

30.

30. Thigh Kneading

**a. First focusing on one hand, gently squeeze with your thumb opposite your fingers. While squeezing, slide a few inches in the direction of your other hand. Next release your squeeze.**

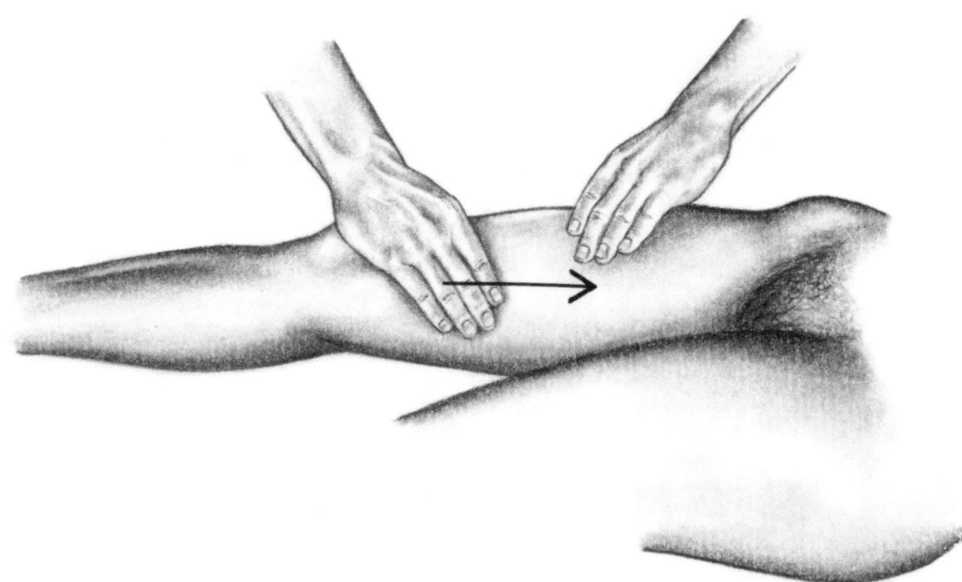

**b. Then, follow the same pattern with the other hand.**

**Gradually knead the entire front thigh.**

Repeat #28

31.

31. Repeat:
Front-Of-Leg Connecting Stroke (#28).

\- - -

**Continue with the right foot before massaging the left leg.**

Ankle Circling

32.

# FEET

Instruction: Written as applied to the right foot.

## 32. Ankle Circling

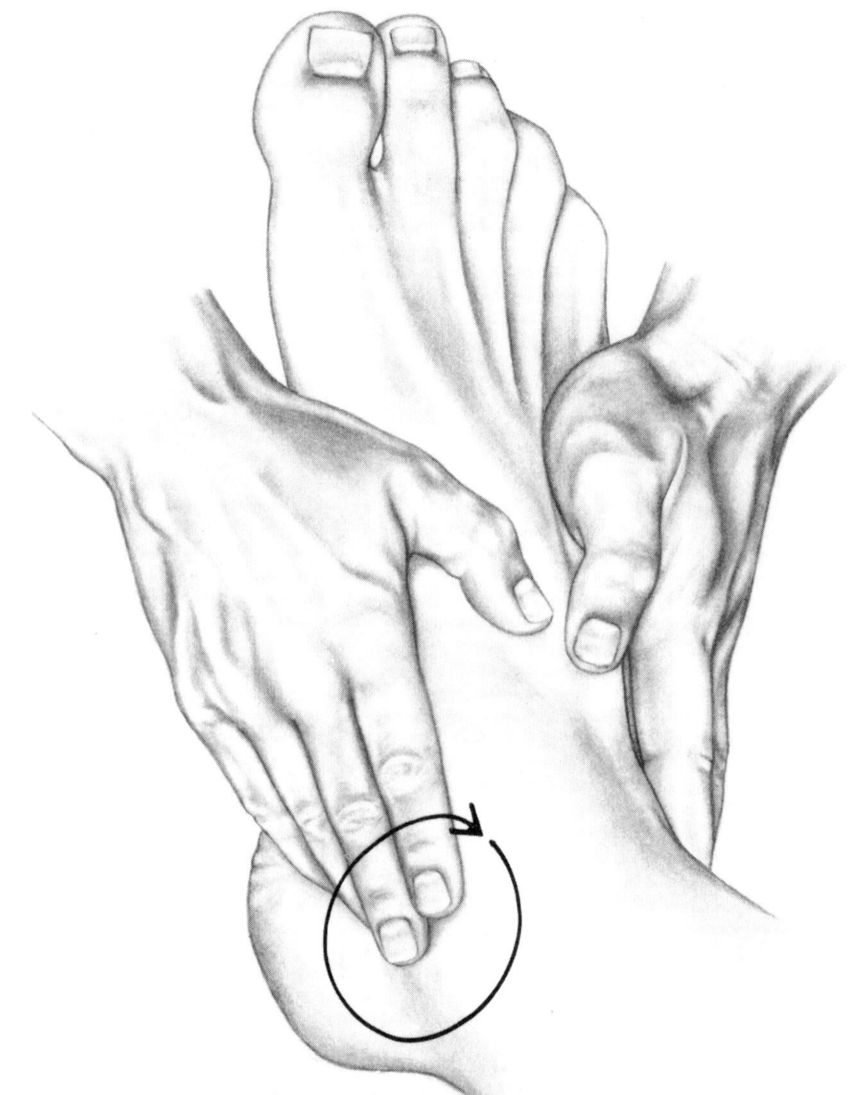

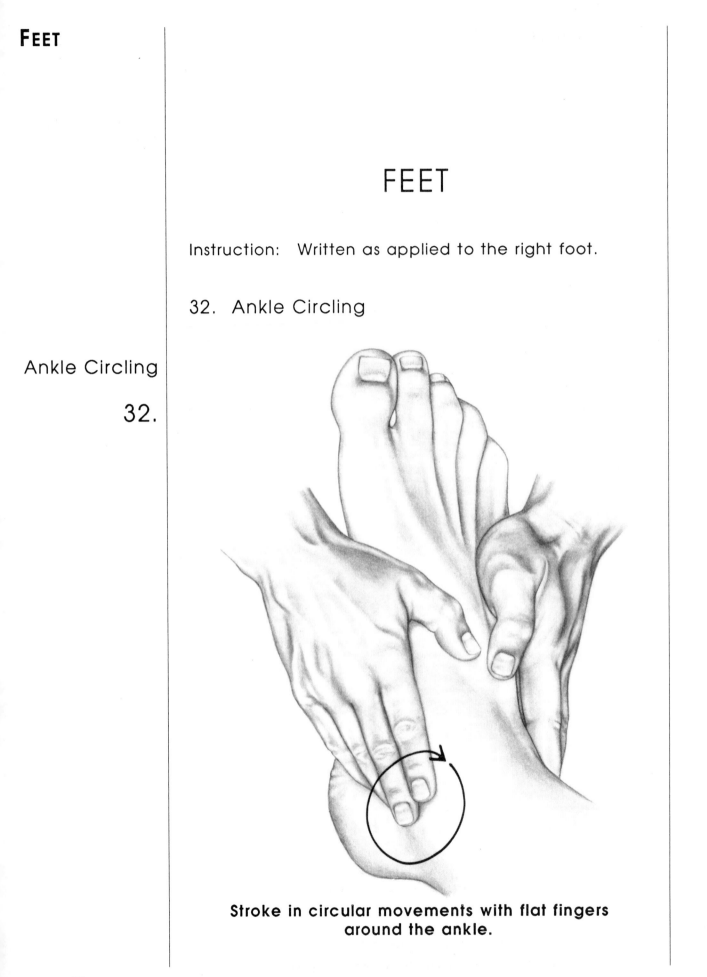

**Stroke in circular movements with flat fingers around the ankle.**

## 33. Connecting Stroke

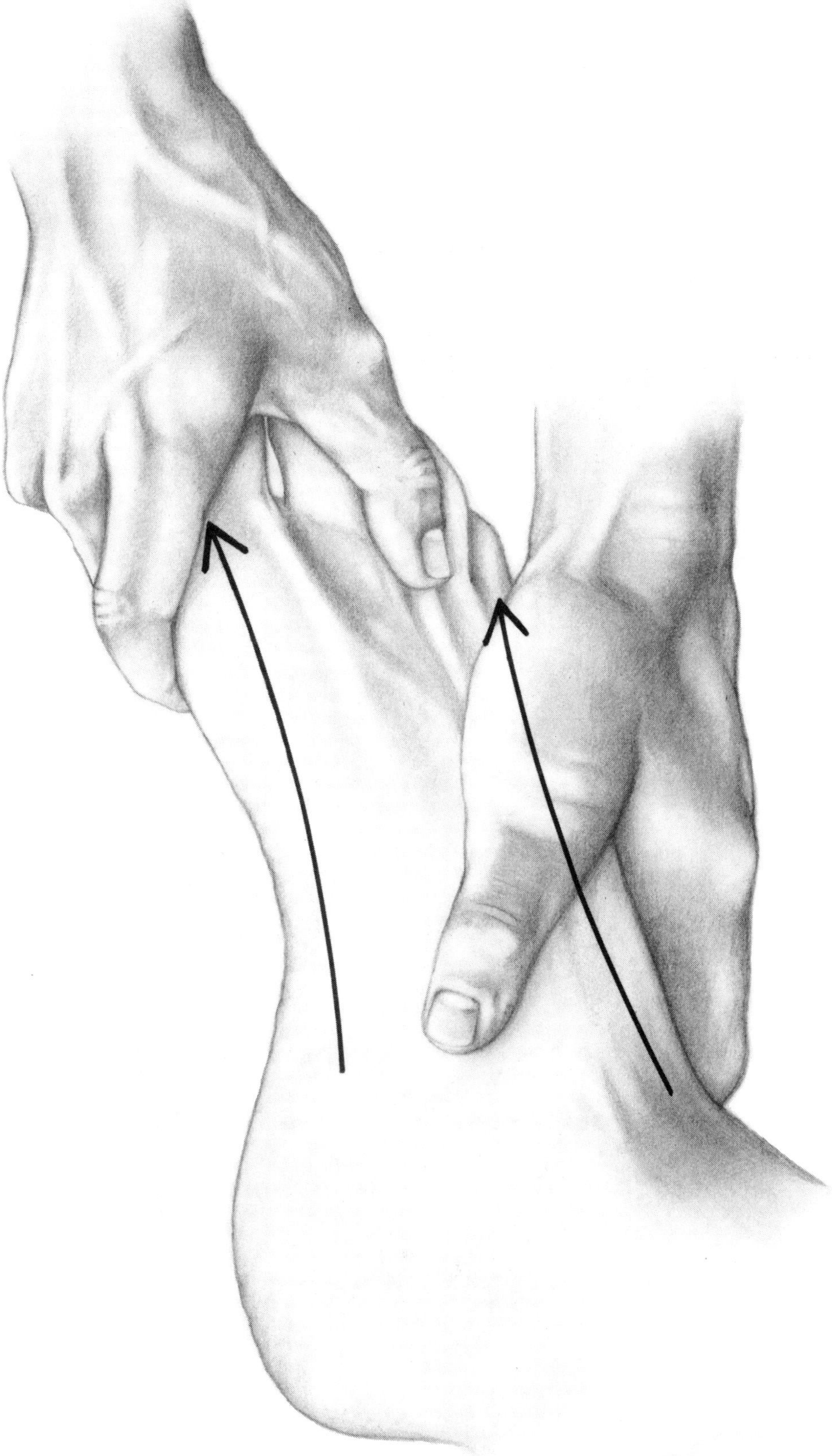

**Alternating your hands, squeeze the foot and slide off the end.**

**Repeat this stroke several times.**

Arc de Triomphe

34.

## 34. Arc de Triomphe

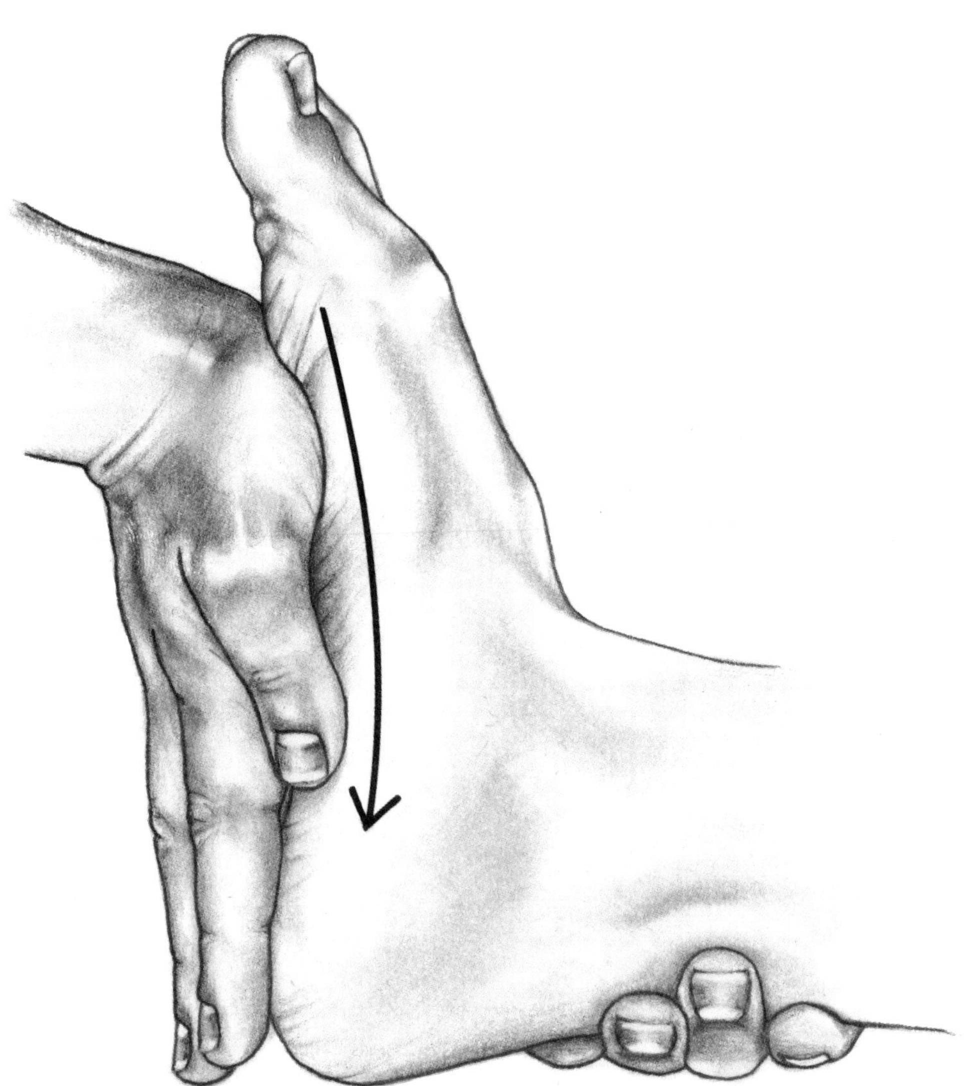

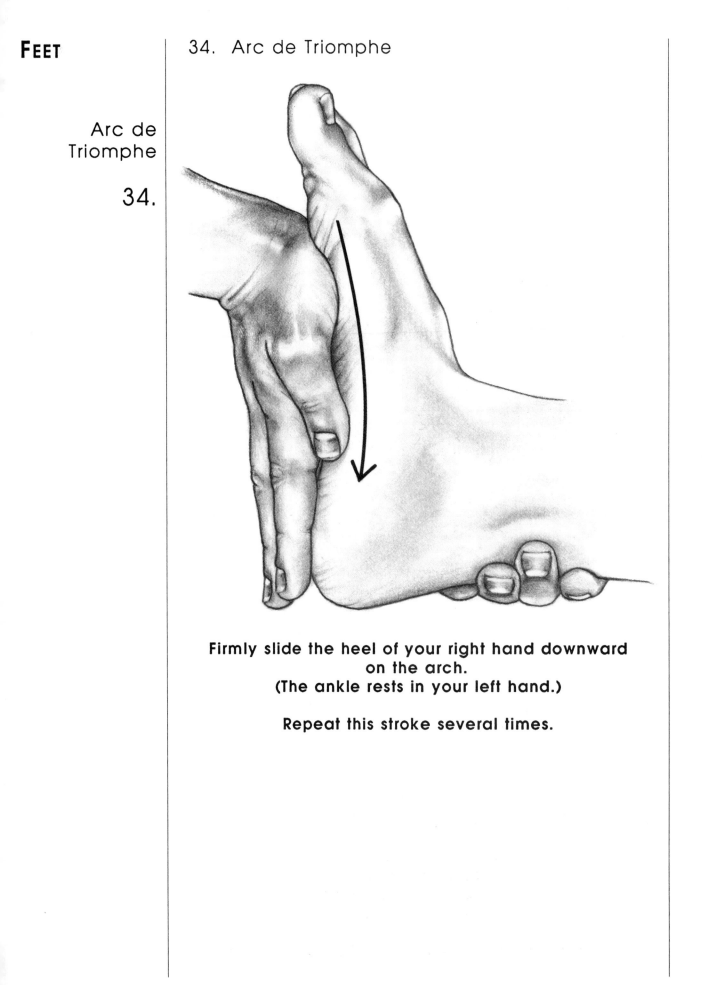

**Firmly slide the heel of your right hand downward on the arch.**
**(The ankle rests in your left hand.)**

**Repeat this stroke several times.**

## 35. Finger Circles

Finger Circles

35.

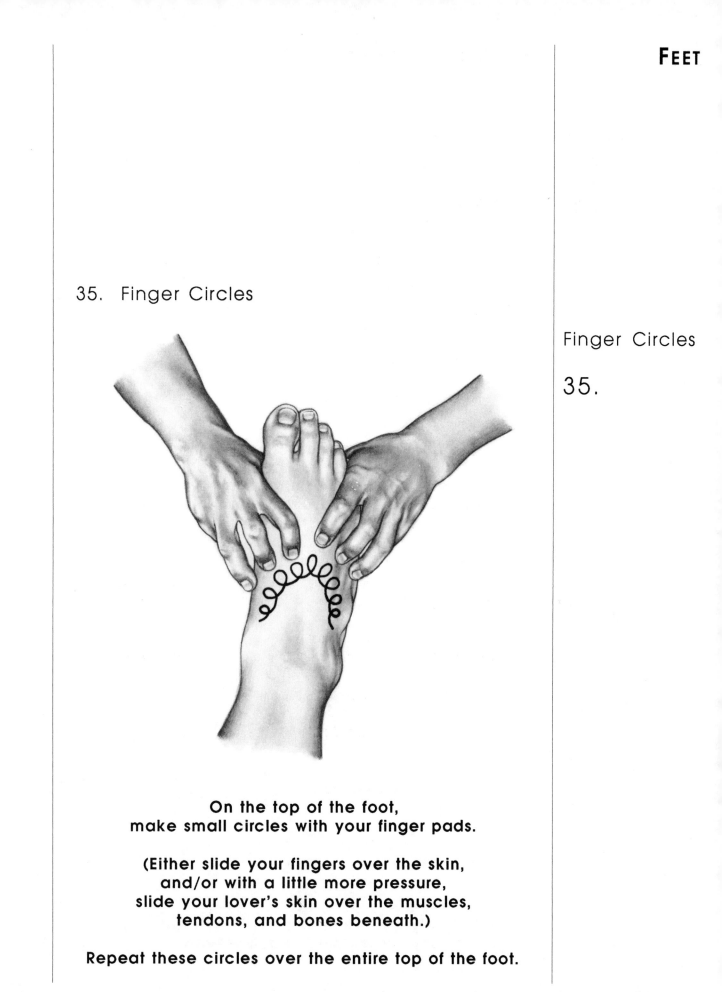

**On the top of the foot,
make small circles with your finger pads.**

**(Either slide your fingers over the skin,
and/or with a little more pressure,
slide your lover's skin over the muscles,
tendons, and bones beneath.)**

**Repeat these circles over the entire top of the foot.**

Between-The-Toes Stroke

36.

## 36. Between-The-Toes Stroke

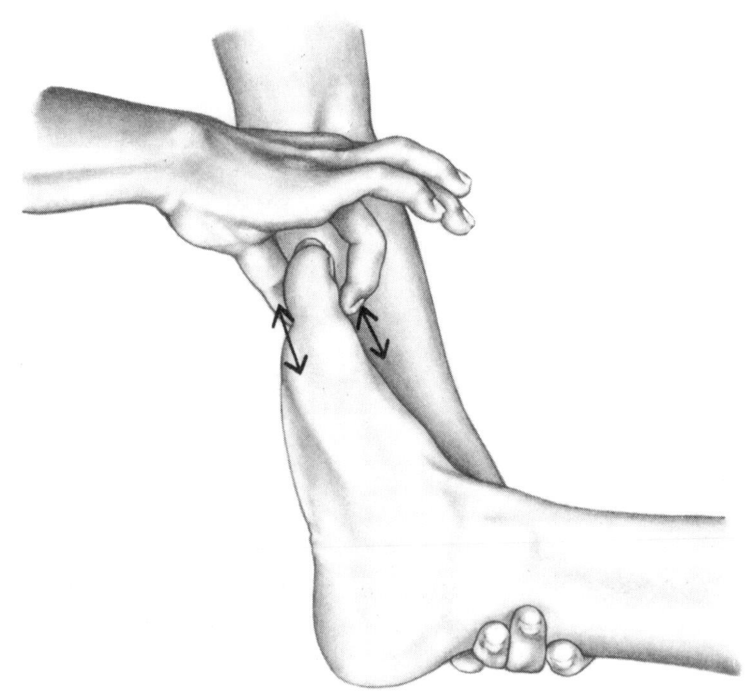

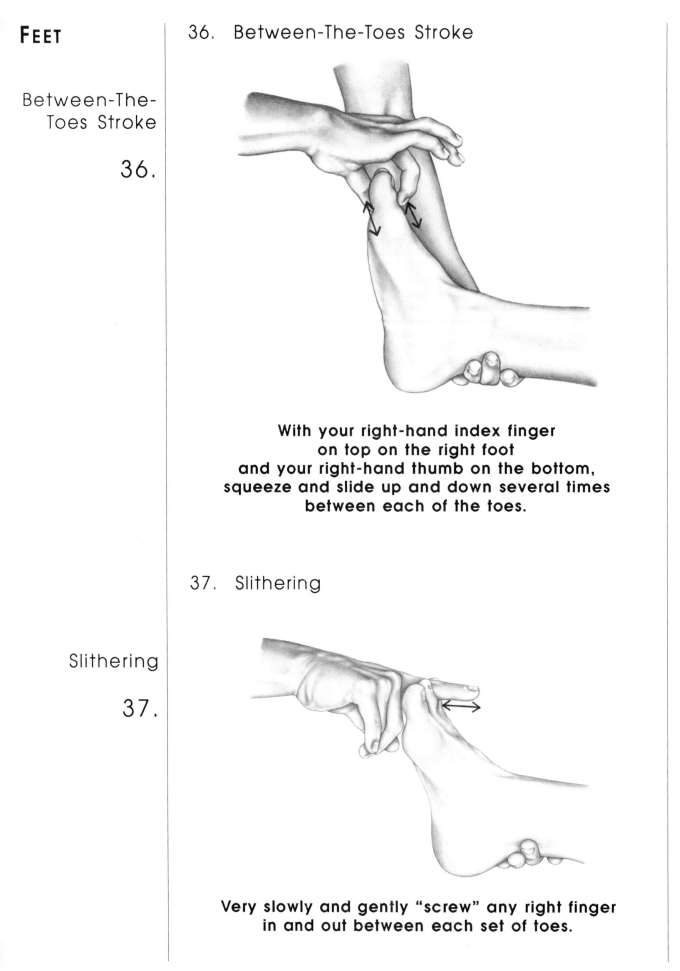

**With your right-hand index finger on top on the right foot and your right-hand thumb on the bottom, squeeze and slide up and down several times between each of the toes.**

Slithering

37.

## 37. Slithering

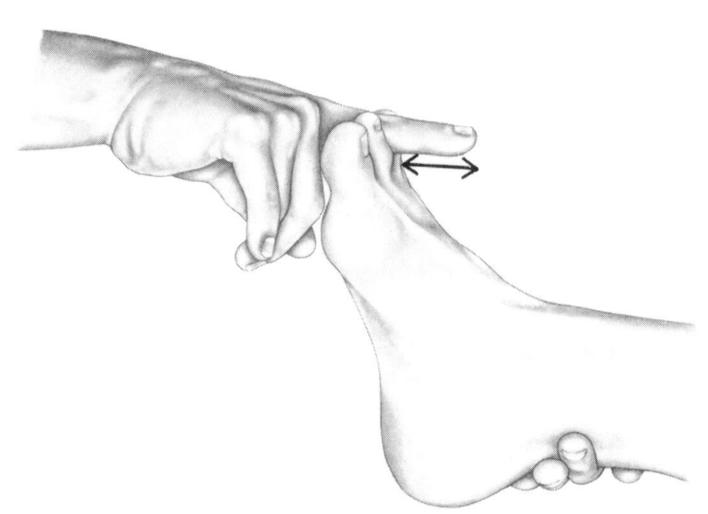

**Very slowly and gently "screw" any right finger in and out between each set of toes.**

38. Repeat:
Front-Of-Leg Connecting Stroke (#28)

Repeat #28
38.

39. Leg and Foot Feather Stroke

**Alternating your hands in a pulling movement, delicately stroke your fingertips over the entire leg and foot — sometimes short strokes, sometimes long ones.**

Feather Stroke
39.

40. Follow the same Front-Of-Legs and Feet sequence on the left side.

**Remember to reverse your right- and left-hand positions.**

Same Front-Of-Legs and Feet Sequence on Left Side
40.

# FRONT TORSO

Your Position: Initially at your lover's right side.

## 41. Moon Stroke

Moon Stroke: practice

41.

**First, practice your right- and left-hand movements separately:**

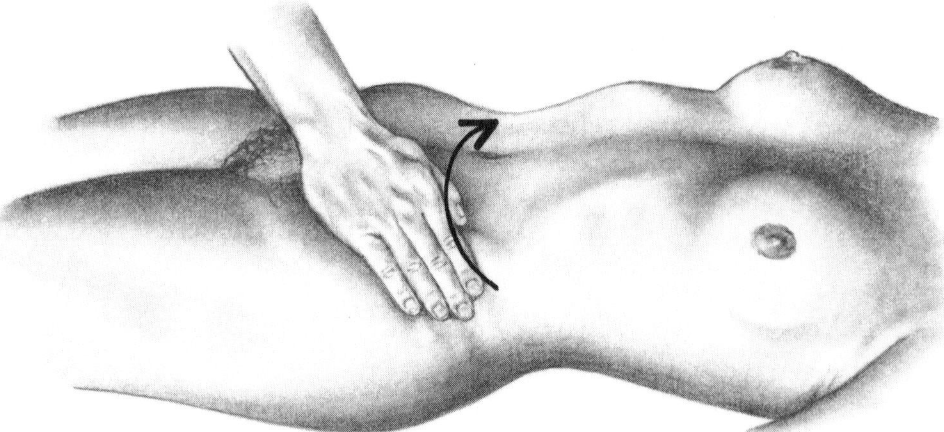

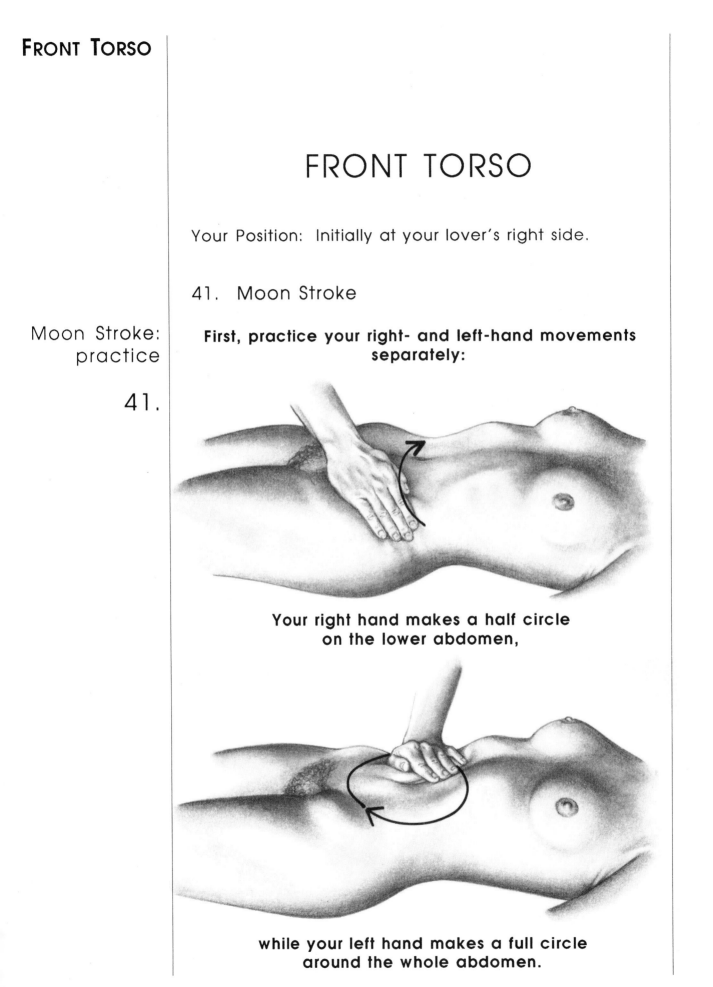

**Your right hand makes a half circle on the lower abdomen,**

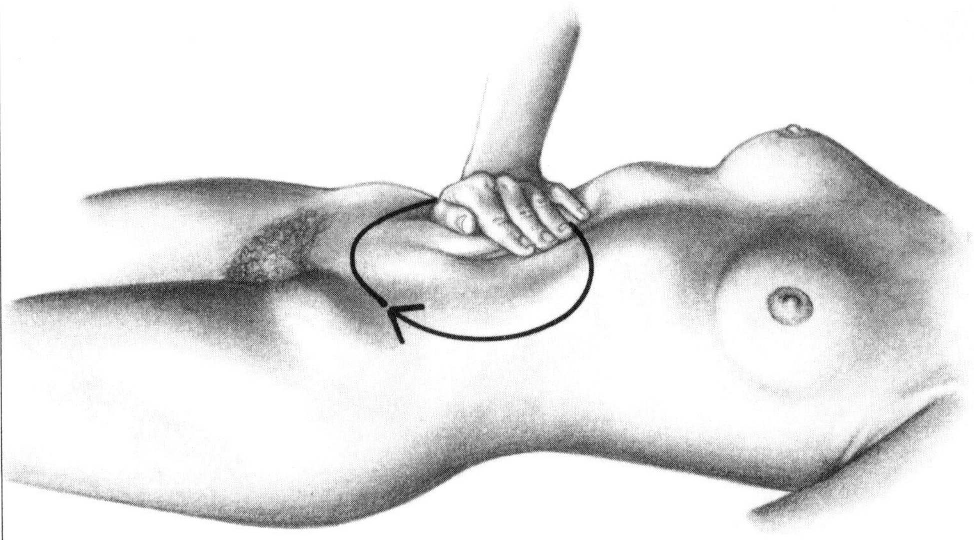

**while your left hand makes a full circle around the whole abdomen.**

Moon Stroke: complete version

41.

This is the complete version:

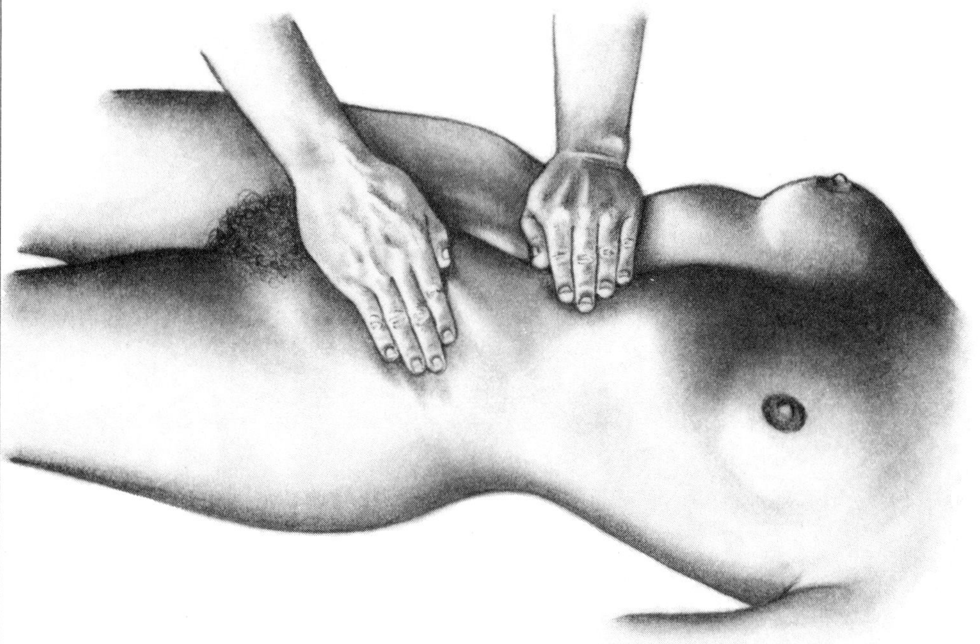

Coordinate your hand movements:
when your right hand is stroking in a half circle,
your left hand is directly opposite on the circle.

When not using your right hand,
simply lift it out of the way
of your left hand's full-circle pattern.

Repeat this whole stroke several times.

42. Center Slide

Center Slide

42.

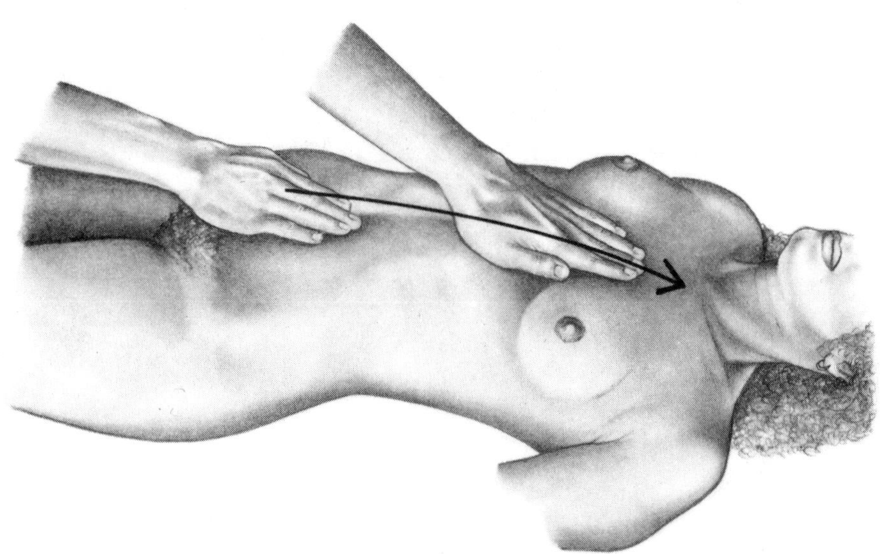

Alternating your hands,
firmly and slowly slide them up the midline
from the lower abdomen to the upper chest.

## 43. Breast Kneading

Instructions: Written as applied to the right breast.

Breast Kneading

43. A

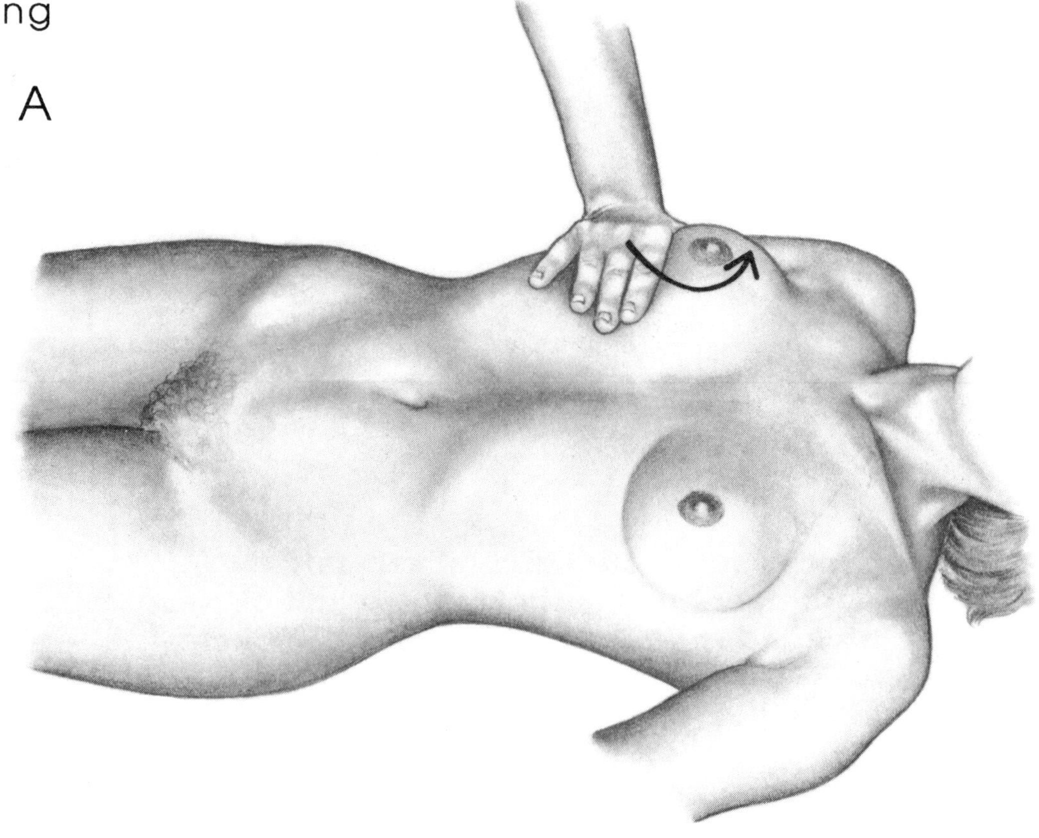

**A.**

**Starting at the lower, outer side of the breast area, slide your right hand up over the breast so that your thumb and index finger encircle the nipple.**

**Using the nipple as the axis, continue the stroke by rotating your hand counterclockwise around the nipple as you slide up and off the breast.**

## Breast Kneading

## 43. B

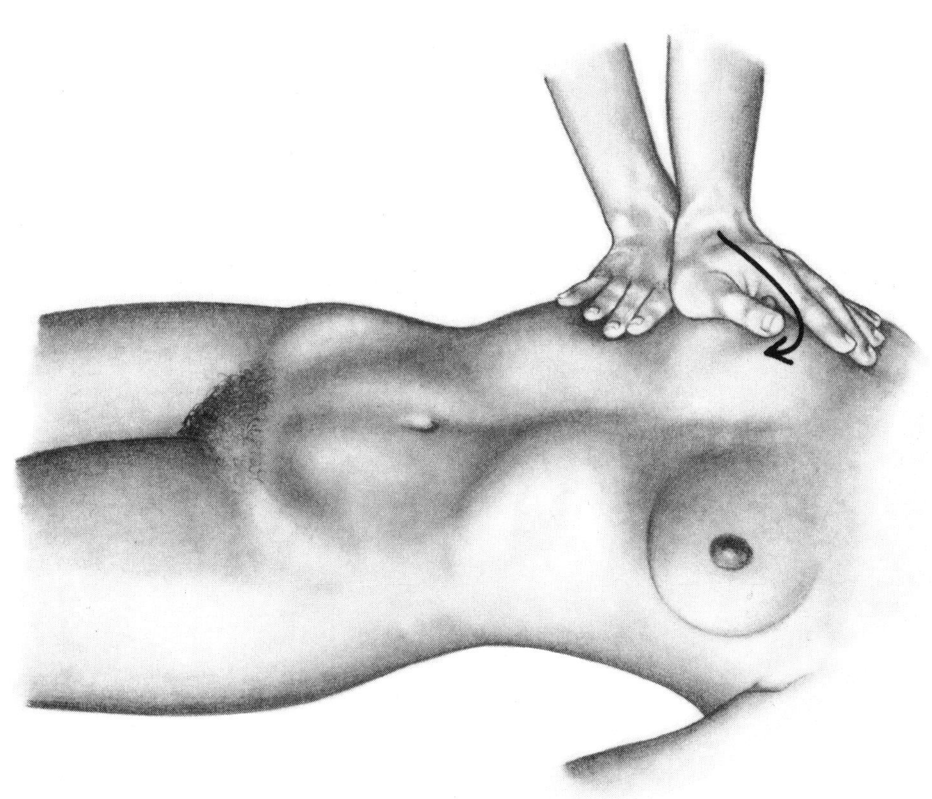

**B.**

**Slide your left hand
from the same lower, outer side of the breast area
up over the breast
so that your thumb and index finger
encircle the nipple.**

**Using the nipple as the axis,
continue the stroke
by rotating your left hand clockwise
around the nipple
as you slide up and off the breast.**

**- - -**

**Repeat this series (A-B) several times
with one hand following the other.**

**- - -**

**Continue with the following stroke (#44)
on the right breast
before massaging the left breast.**

**Note:**
**On a woman's breast, apply a lighter pressure.**

Spokes Stroke

44. A

## 44. Spokes Stroke

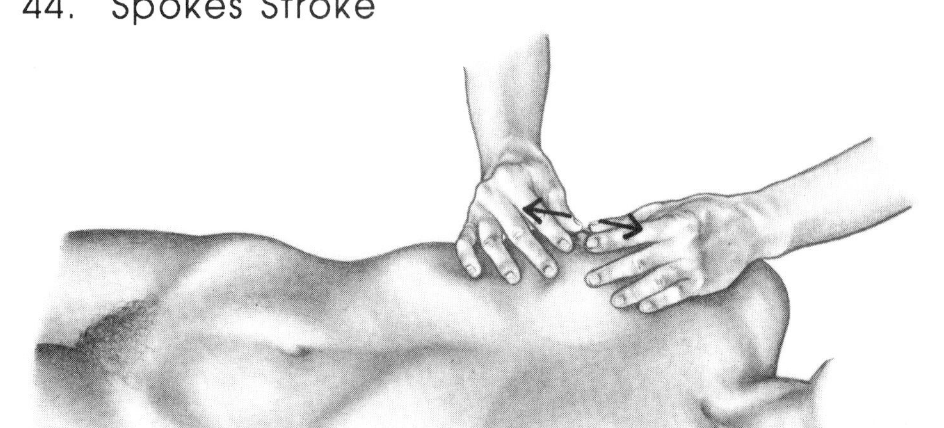

A.
Imagine the nipple as the axis in a wheel
with spokes radiating out from the axis.
Using the pads of the fingers and thumbs
of both hands,
gently squeeze at the axis
and slide out along a spoke,
moving your hands in opposite directions.

Repeat this pattern several times
along the different spokes.

44. B

B.
Gently squeeze the base of the nipple
between the pads
of your index finger and thumb
of one hand
and slide UP and off the nipple.
Follow this pattern,
alternating your hands
one immediately after the other.

Now move to the other side
and repeat this and the previous stroke
(#43 and #44)
on the other breast area.

## 45. Side Pulling

Side Pulling

45. A

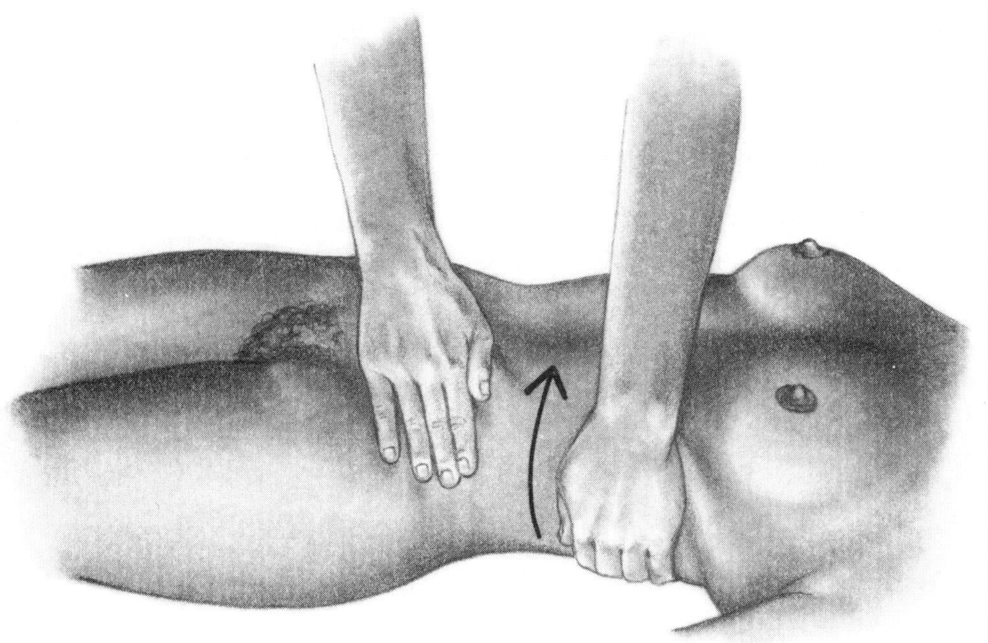

**A.**
**Alternating your hands, slide them in a pulling manner across the side of the torso toward the front midline.**

**(This series includes the area from the hips to near the underarms. Be gentle on the mammary area.)**

45. B

**B.**
**Move to the other side, and apply the pulling movements to the opposite side.**

## 46. Torso Feather Stroke

Torso Feather Stroke

46.

**Alternating your hands in a pulling movement, delicately stroke your fingertips over the entire torso. Include the genital and thigh areas as well.**

# GENITALS: MALE

Lover's Position: Lying on back.
Your Position: To your lover's right side.
Note: If you wish to follow safer-sex practices, please consult the appendix.

## 47. Sweet Thrills

Sweet Thrills

47. A

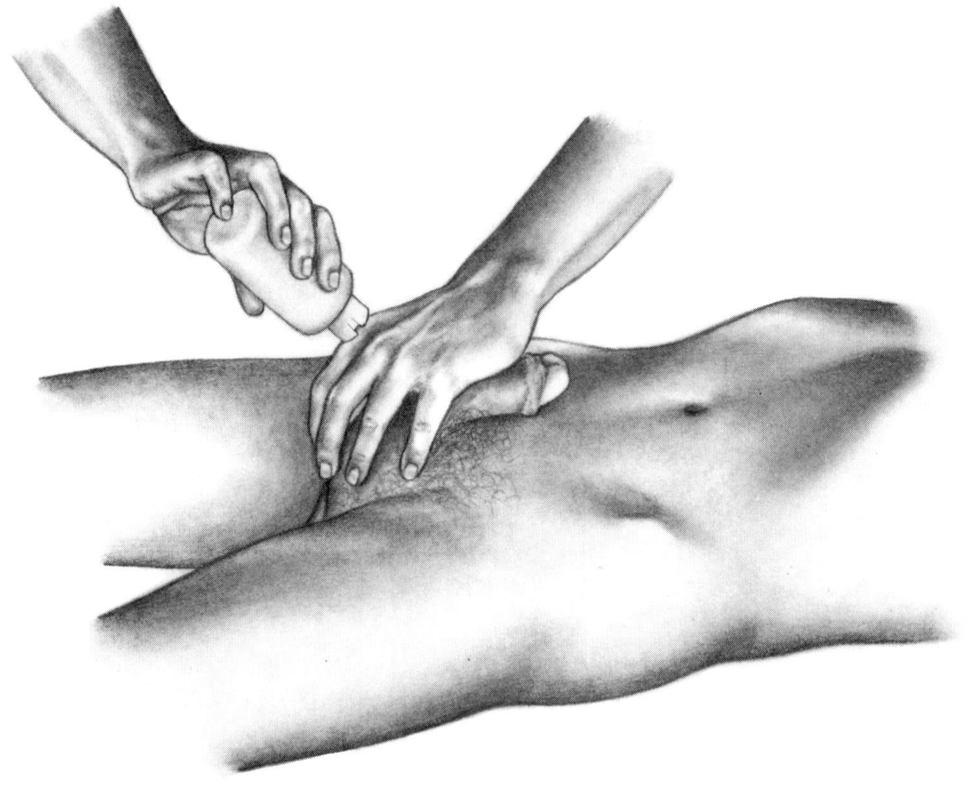

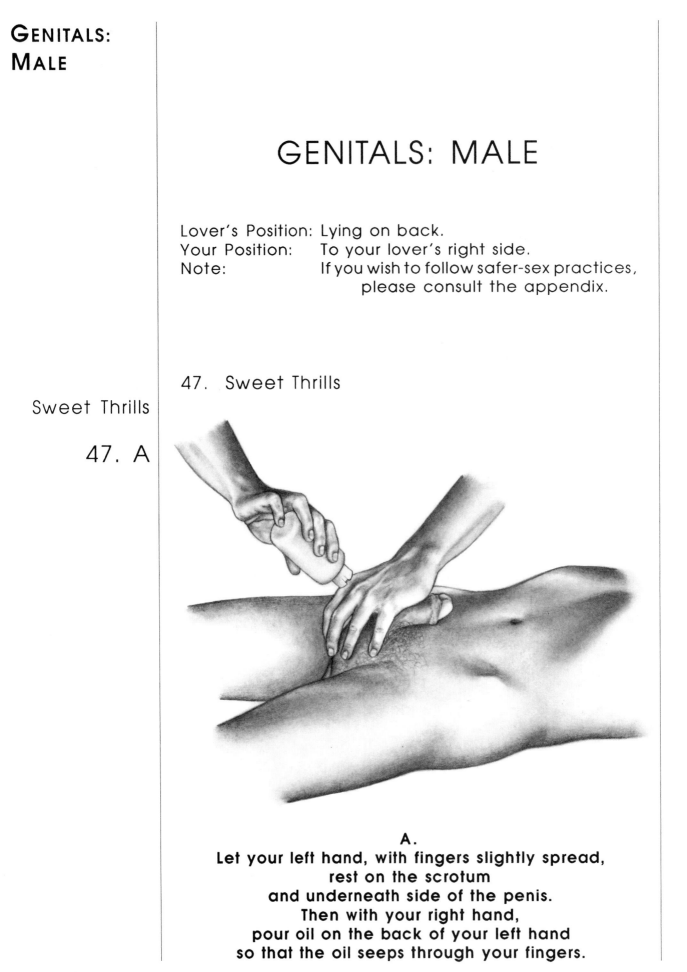

**A.**
**Let your left hand, with fingers slightly spread,
rest on the scrotum
and underneath side of the penis.
Then with your right hand,
pour oil on the back of your left hand
so that the oil seeps through your fingers.**

## 47. B

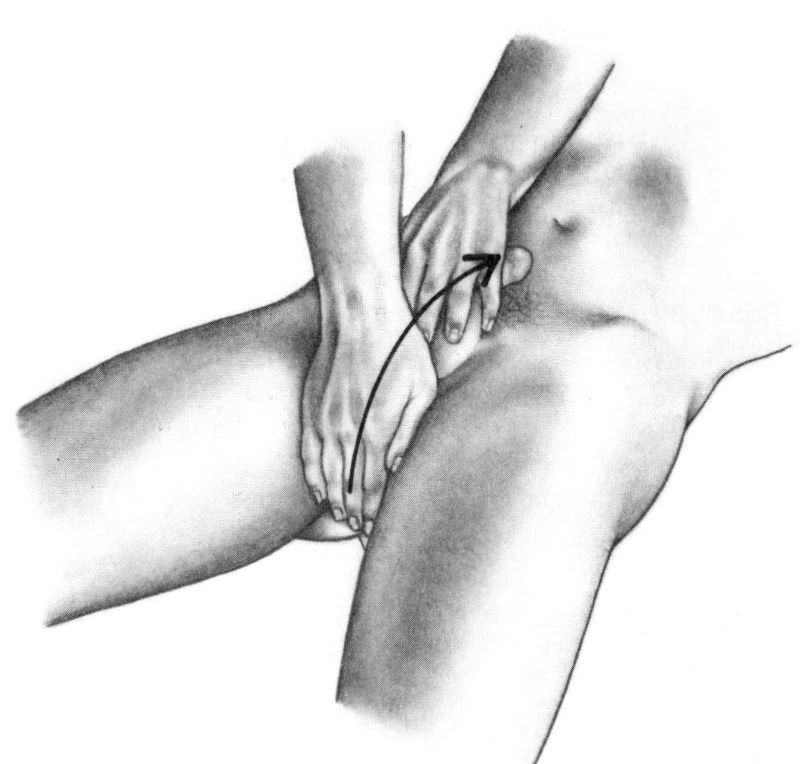

**B.**
**Alternating your hands,
spread the oil with a pulling up motion,
sliding from the pelvic floor up
over the scrotum and penis.**

**Perhaps give a little firmer pressure
on the pelvic floor.**

**Be sure there is plenty of oil
since the following strokes
assume well-lubricated motions.**

Note: Should your lover ejaculate during this or any other stroke, perhaps go to "Being," #58.

The Juicer

48.

## 48. The Juicer

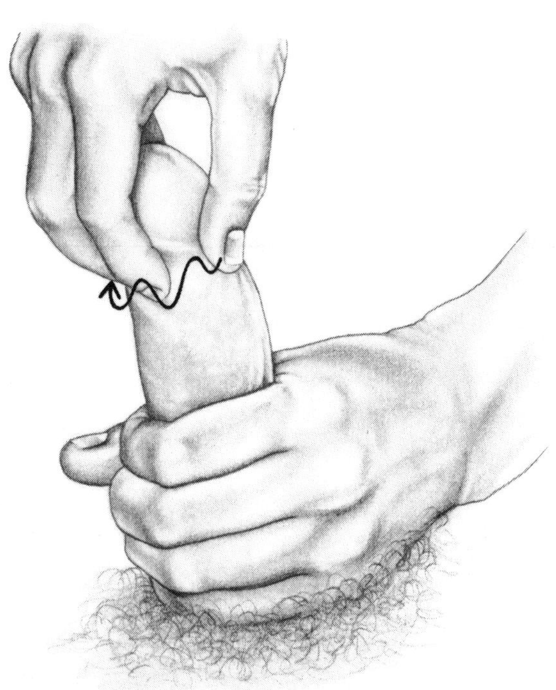

**Your left hand gently stretches the foreskin down along the shaft of the flaccid or erect penis.**

**Your right hand points
as if to twist a halved orange on a juicer.
Concentrating on the head of the penis,
rotate your right-hand fingers back and forth
in coordination with an up-and-down sliding motion.**

**Vary the amount of pressure from your right hand.**

## 49. The Snake

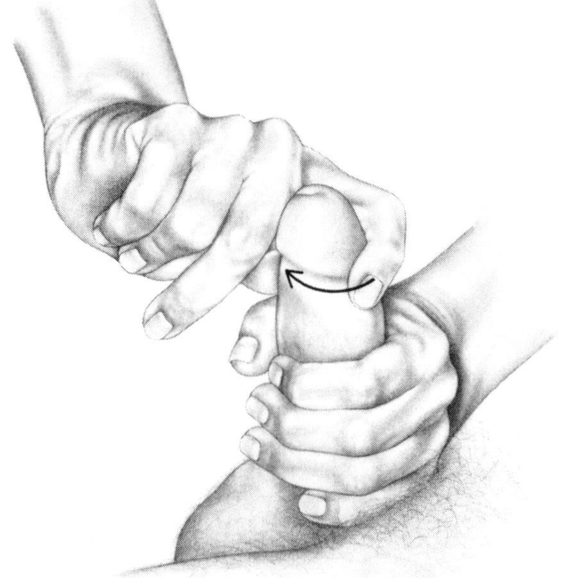

The Snake

49. a

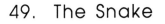

a: Your left hand gently stretches the foreskin down along the shaft of the flaccid or erect penis.

Your right thumb and index finger form a snug circle just below the head of the penis and rotate in a clockwise direction as far as your wrist permits.

49. b

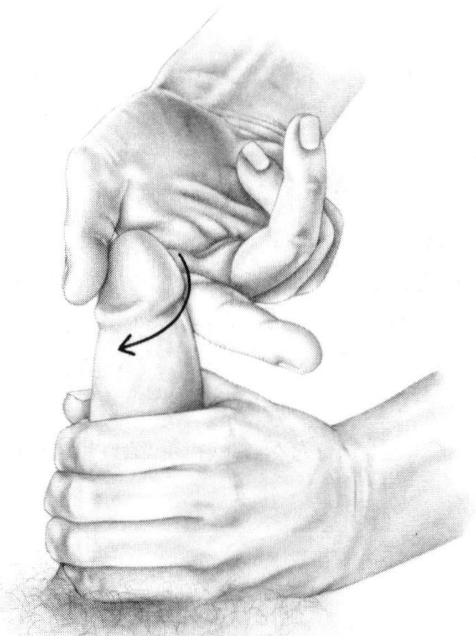

b: Continuing the movement, lift your right thumb so that your index finger can maintain contact in the rotation until the thumb can form a circle with the index finger again.

Repeat this circling several times.

Countdown

50.

## 50. Countdown

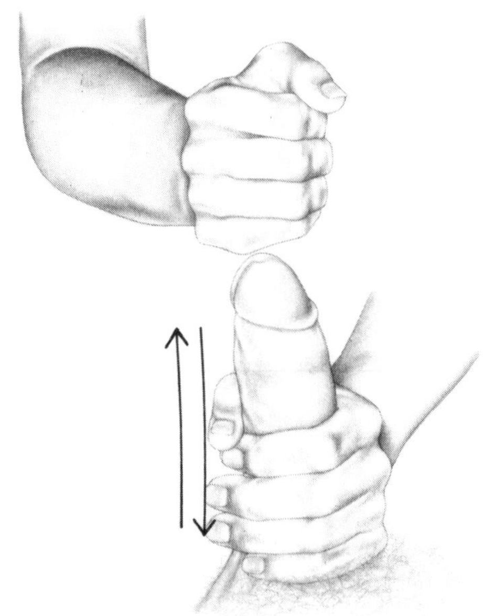

**Using plenty of oil and alternating your hands,
make ten downward strokes
on the flaccid or erect penis,
then ten upward strokes.
Follow with nine downward, nine upward,
eight downward, eight upward
— all the way to one down and one up.**

**Suggestion:
syncopate the rhythm of your stroking.
Rather than using an even beat (1-2-3-4-5-6),
wait a moment after each set of two strokes
(1-2—3-4—5-6).**

## 51. The Scrotum Ring



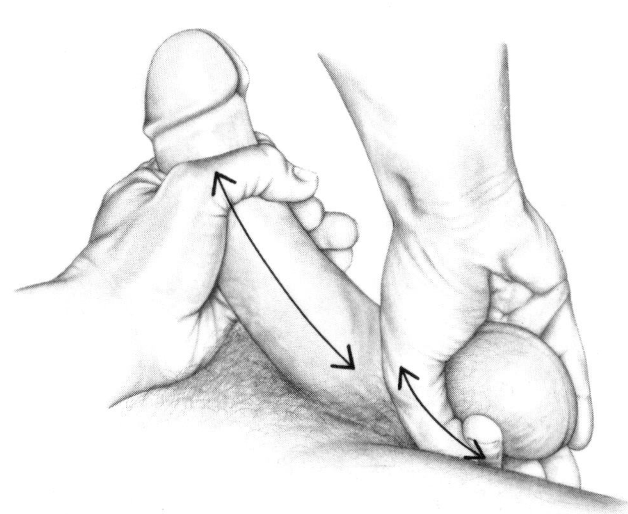

**Your right thumb along with your index and perhaps middle fingers encircle the scrotum between the base of the penis and the testicles. (Be careful not to squeeze the testicles.)**

**Now move the scrotum up and down as your left hand strokes up and down on the flaccid or erect penile shaft.**

**Vary the amount of pressure of your right hand against the base of the penis.**

**- - -**

**To continue the Male Genital strokes, go to "Feelin' Good All Over," #57, which is for both men and women.**

# GENITALS: FEMALE

Lover's Position: Lying on back.
Your Position: To your lover's right side.
Note: Be certain your fingernails are smooth and short and your hands are clean when massaging membranous tissues areas.
Note: If you wish to follow safer-sex practices, please consult the appendix.

## 52. Sweet Thrills

Sweet Thrills

52. A

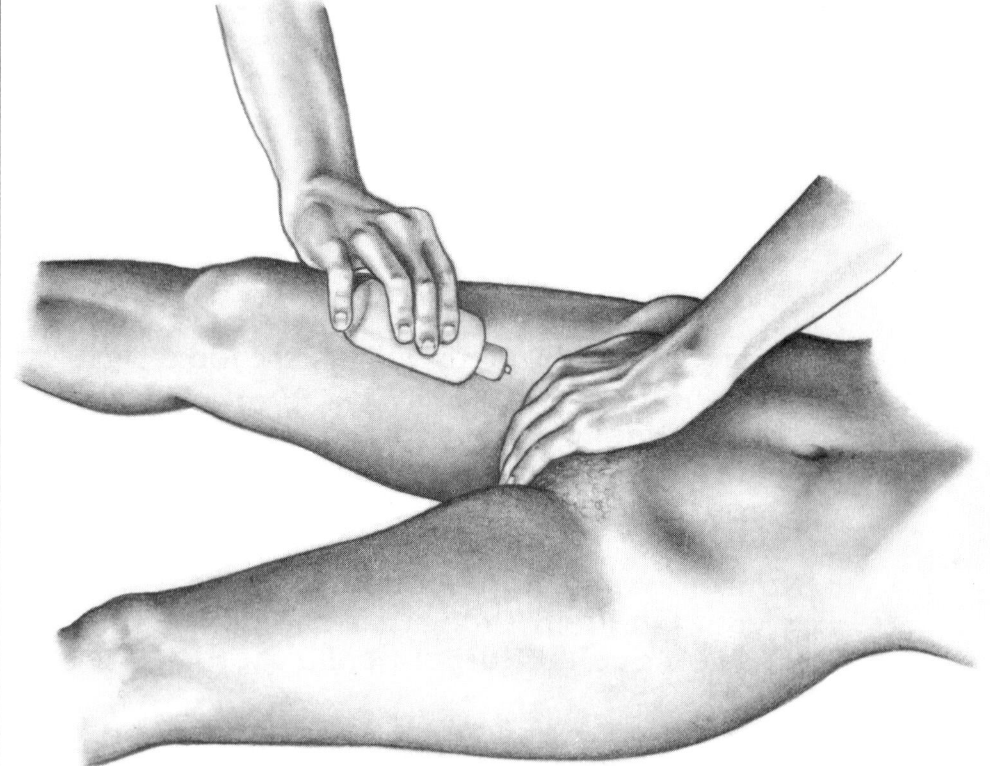

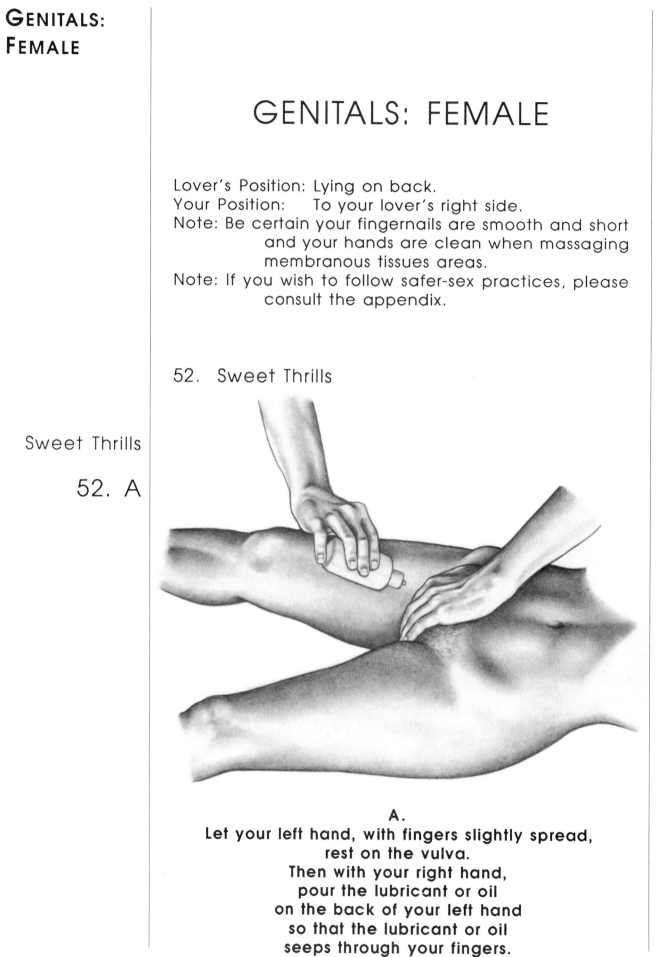

**A.**
**Let your left hand, with fingers slightly spread, rest on the vulva. Then with your right hand, pour the lubricant or oil on the back of your left hand so that the lubricant or oil seeps through your fingers.**

Sweet Thrills

52. B

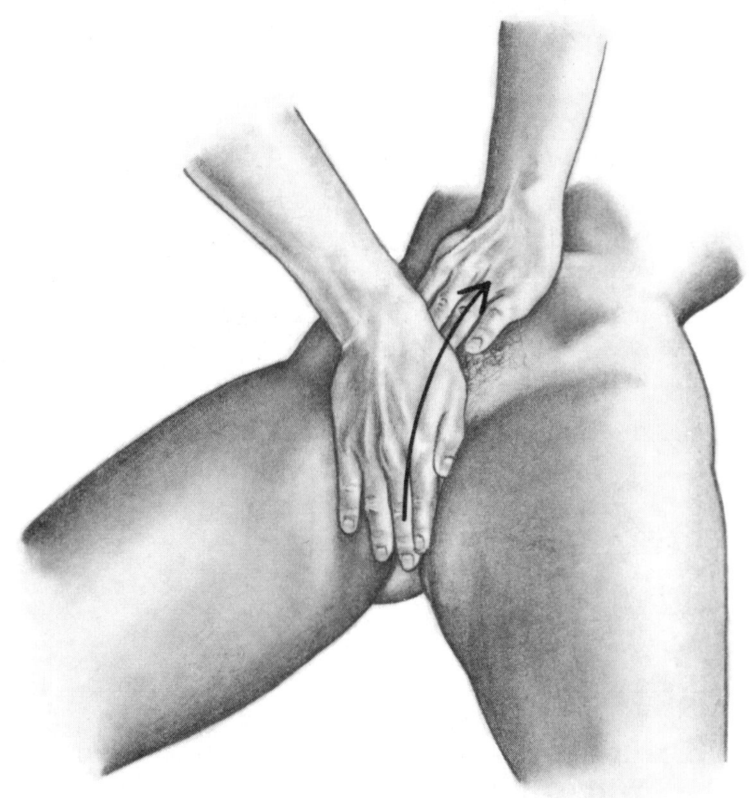

**B.**
**Alternating your hands, spread the lubricant or oil with a pulling up motion by sliding from the lower part of the vulva up over the clitoris and pubic area.**

**Note:**
**Be very careful not to stroke from the anal to the vaginal areas.**

Voluptuous Vulva

53.

## 53. Voluptuous Vulva

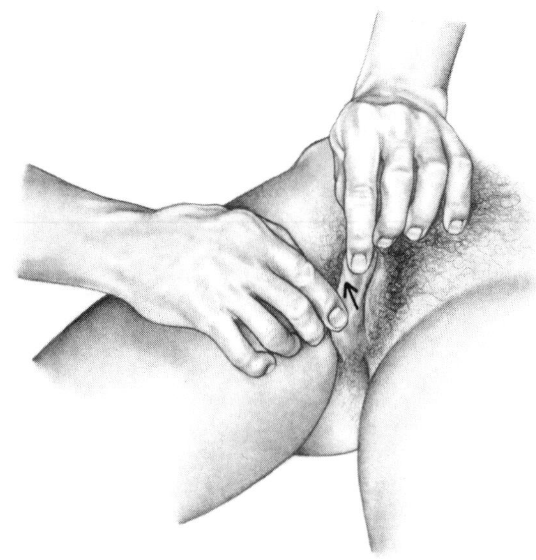

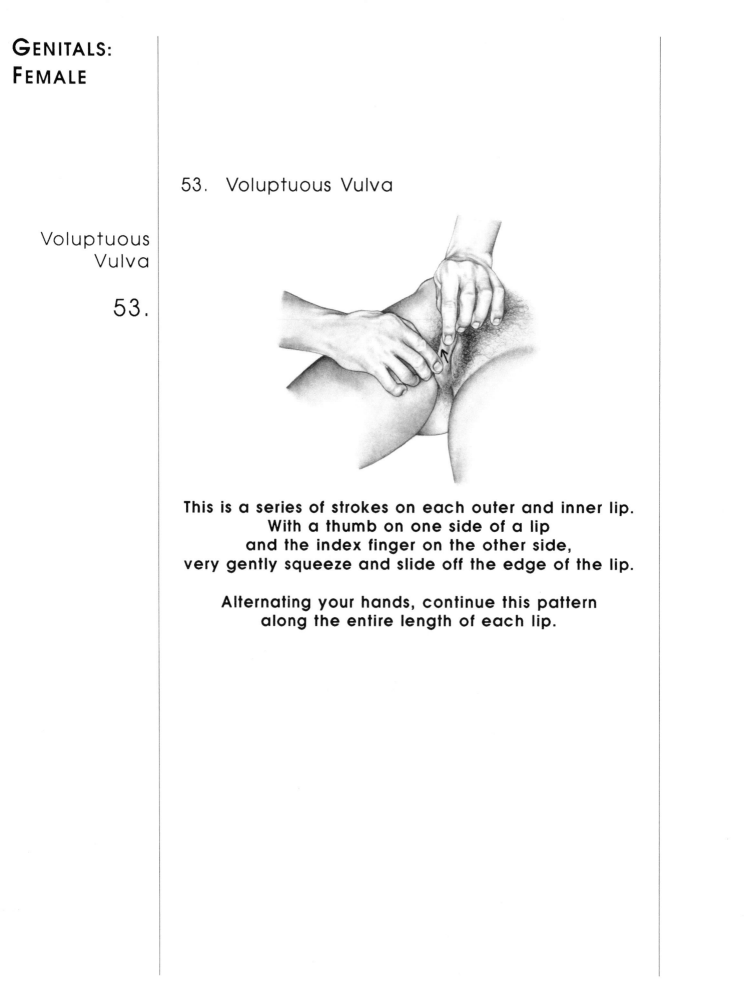

**This is a series of strokes on each outer and inner lip. With a thumb on one side of a lip and the index finger on the other side, very gently squeeze and slide off the edge of the lip.**

**Alternating your hands, continue this pattern along the entire length of each lip.**

## 54. Ring Around The Rosy

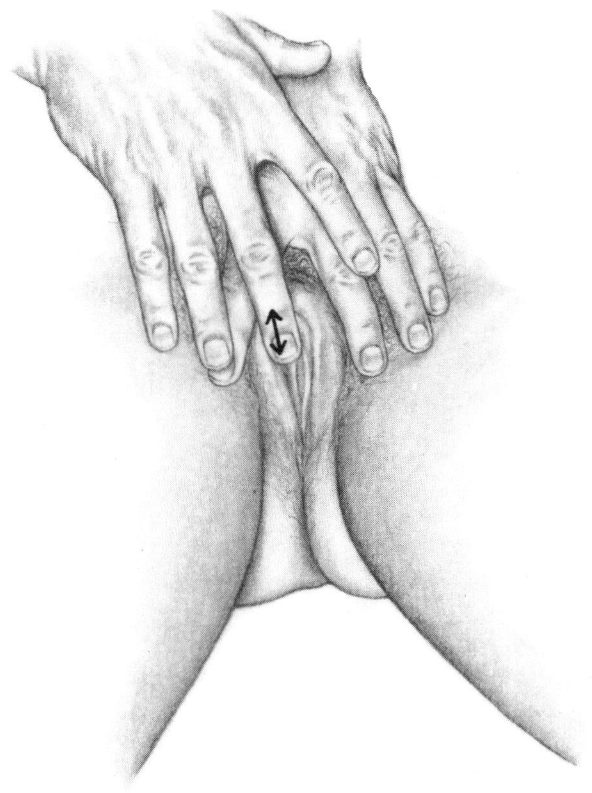

Ring Around The Rosy

54. A

**A.**
**Now you center your stroking around the head of the clitoris, which is just beneath where the inner lips merge together at the upper part of the vulva.**

**To begin, slide the middle finger pad of your right hand up and down several times between the inner and outer lips on one side of the vulva and then on the other side.**

54. B

**B.**
**With one or two fingers, slowly massage circles around the clitoral head, several times in one directions, then several times in the other direction.**

54. C

**C.**
**With a single finger pad, begin a very slow, upward stroke at the vaginal entrance, up through the inner lips, up past the clitoral head. Repeat several times.**

Rockin' Around The Clock

55. A

## 55. Rockin' Around The Clock

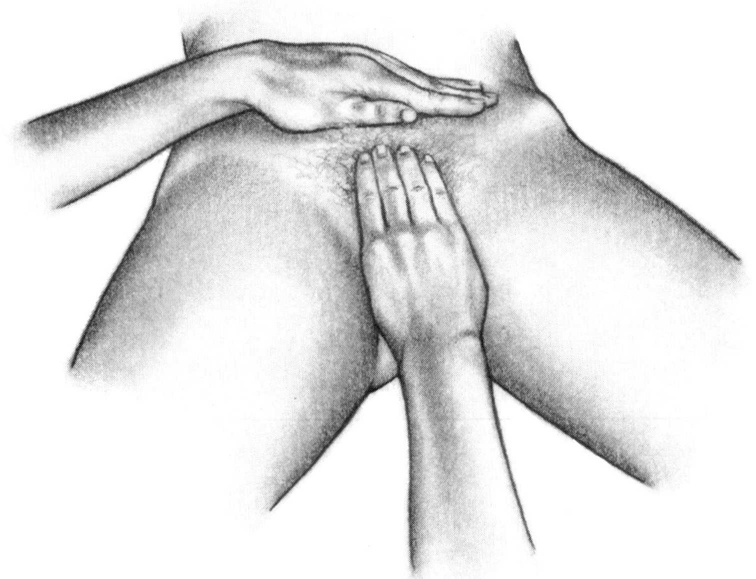

**A.**

**For this intravaginal massage,
imagine a clock at the vaginal entrance,
with twelve o'clock near the clitoris
and six o'clock near the anus.**

**Your left palm rests on the abdomen.
At the twelve-o'clock position
slowly introduce your right thumb into the vagina
until its pad is pressing
upward
on the underneath side
of the pubic bone.**

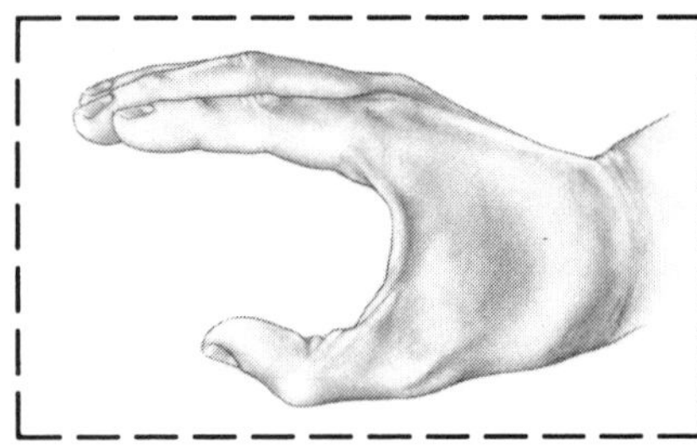

**Now gently rock your right
arm and hand
back and forth about an inch.**

**After about fifteen seconds or longer,
lighten your pressure,
slide your thumb to the one-o'clock position,
and begin to rock again.
Continue in this fashion
until about the seven-o'clock position.**

Rockin' Around The Clock

55. B

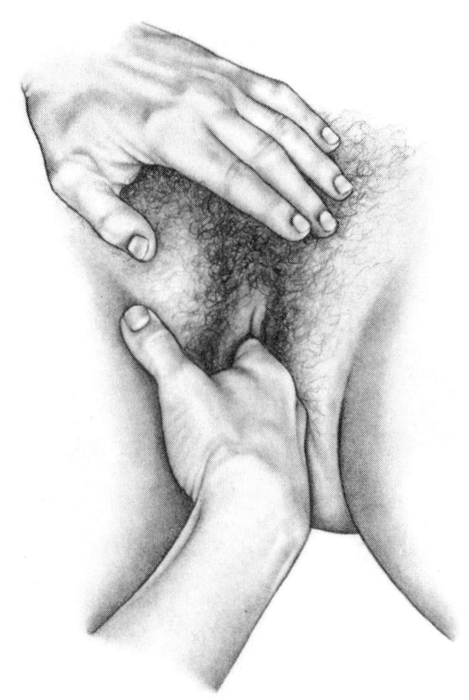

**B.**
**At about seven o'clock, shift to using your index finger and continue with the rocking pattern up through twelve o'clock.**

The Gee!
Stroke

56. A

## 56. The Gee! Stroke

**A.**
**This stroke may be easier if you bring your lover's knees up with both feet resting on the table.**

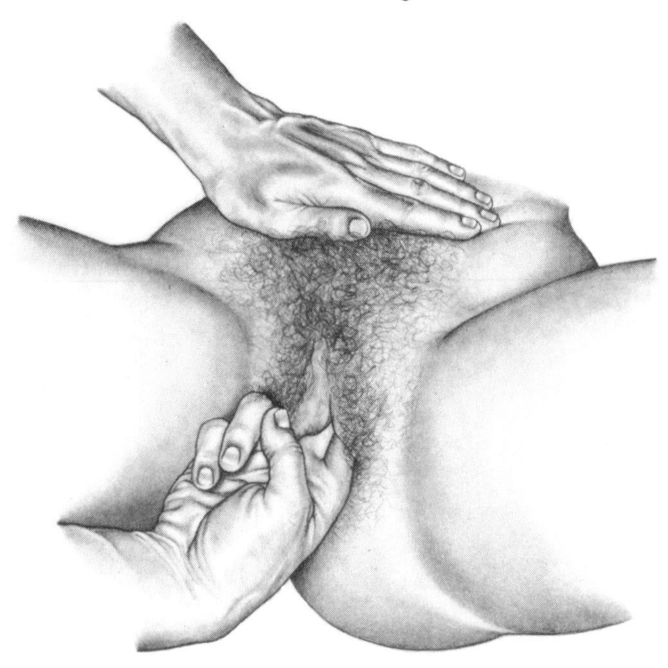

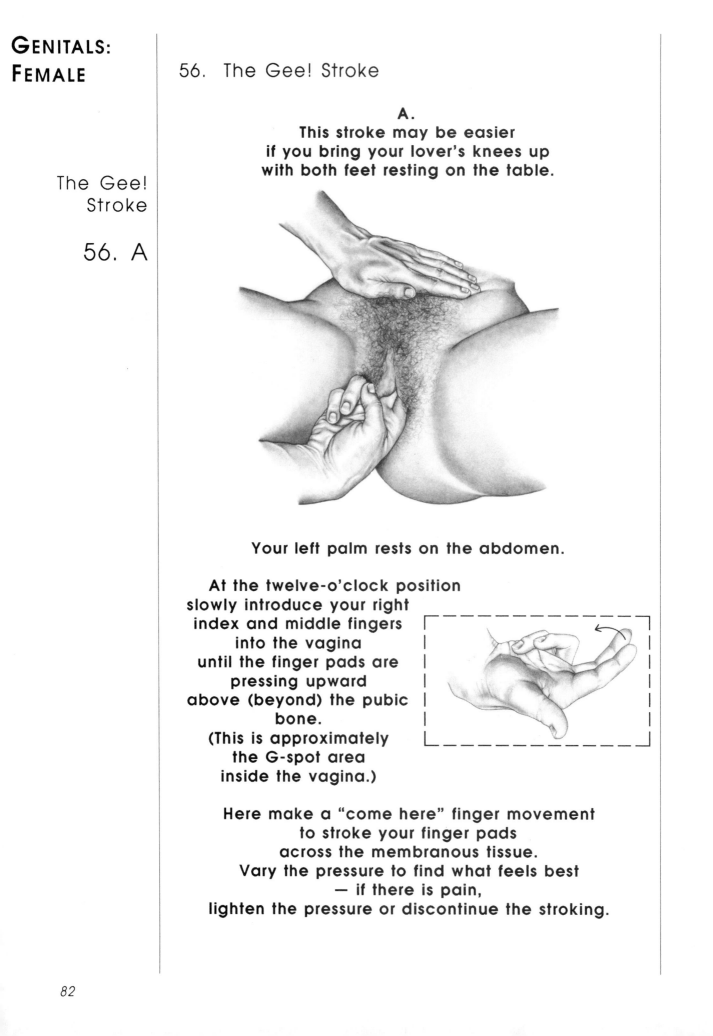

**Your left palm rests on the abdomen.**

**At the twelve-o'clock position slowly introduce your right index and middle fingers into the vagina until the finger pads are pressing upward above (beyond) the pubic bone. (This is approximately the G-spot area inside the vagina.)**

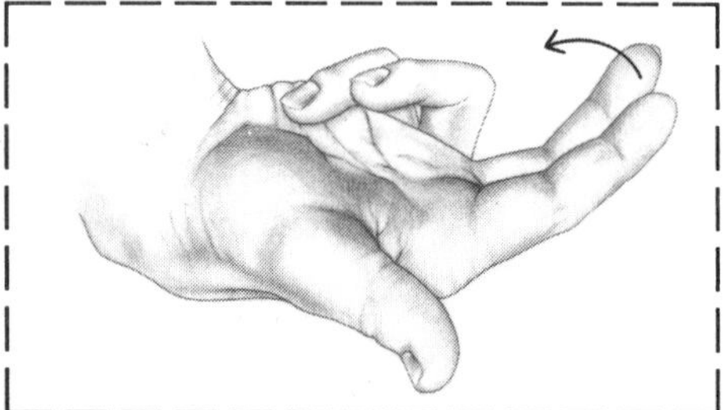

**Here make a "come here" finger movement to stroke your finger pads across the membranous tissue. Vary the pressure to find what feels best — if there is pain, lighten the pressure or discontinue the stroking.**

The Gee! Stroke

56. B

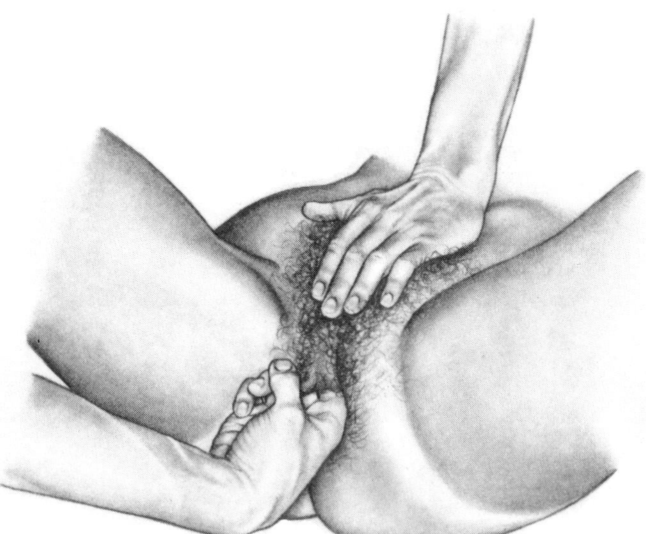

**B.**

**With your right hand continuing Part A, rest the heel of your left hand on the lower abdomen. Now allow your left-hand fingers to delicately stroke the clitoral head at the same time.**

**(Perhaps apply a little pressure on the lower abdomen with the heel of your left hand.)**

**When you complete the stroke, slide your lover's legs back to the flat position.**

**Note: Starting with this stroke, the male and female genital massage description is the same.**

## 57. Feelin' Good All Over

**In this series of strokes
you connect the enjoyable sensations of the genitals
with the enjoyable sensations
of other parts of the body.**

Feelin' Good All Over

57. A

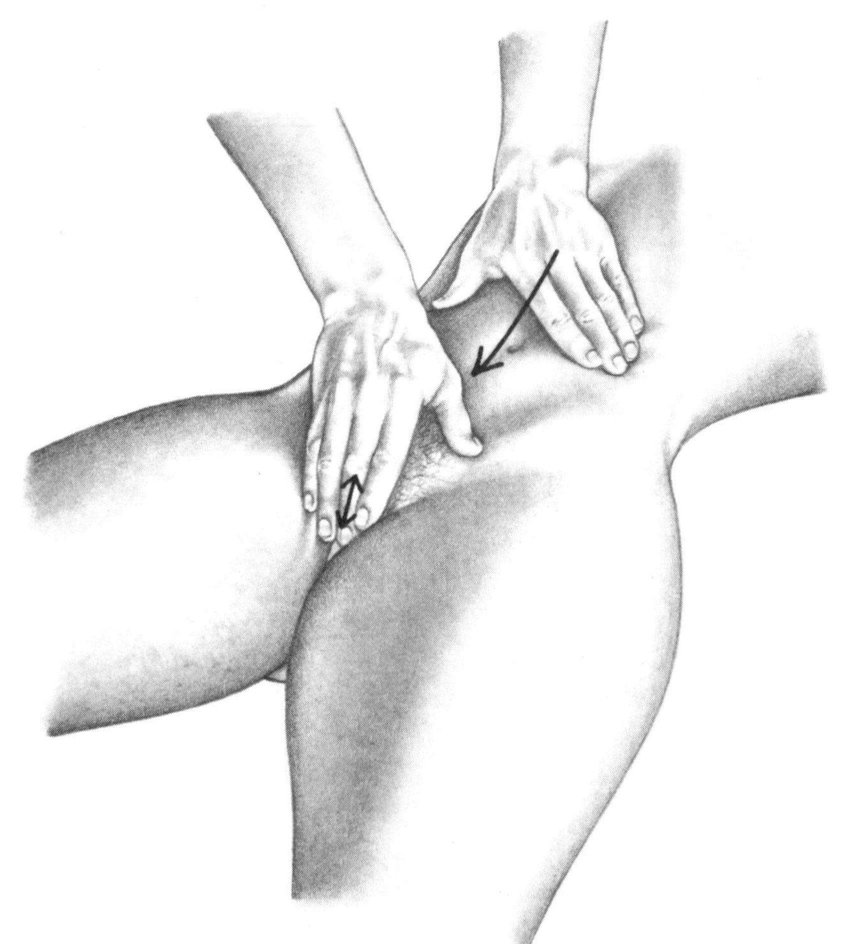

**A. Abdomen and Genitals**

**While your right hand massages the genitals
(in any fashion)
let your left hand knead
or make circular strokes on the abdomen
(For a description of kneading, see stroke #9.)**

57. B

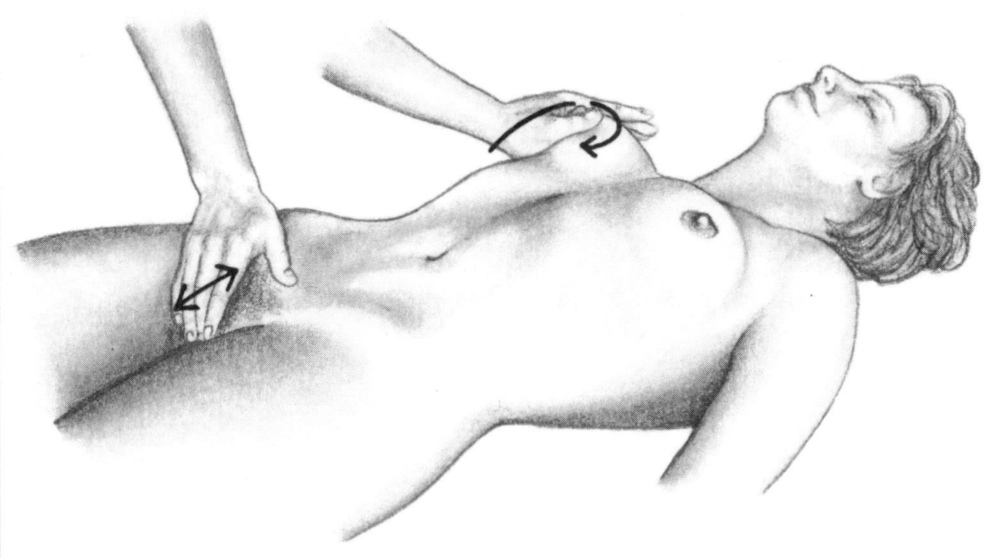

B. Breast Area and Genitals

As your right hand continues as in Part A,
slide your left hand from the same lower, outer side
of the breast area
up over the breast
so that your thumb and index finger
encircle the nipple.
Using the nipple as the axis,
continue the stroke
by rotating your left hand clockwise
around the nipple
as you slide up and off the breast.

Repeat several times on the right breast area
and continue Part C on the right side of the neck
before going to the left side.

57. C

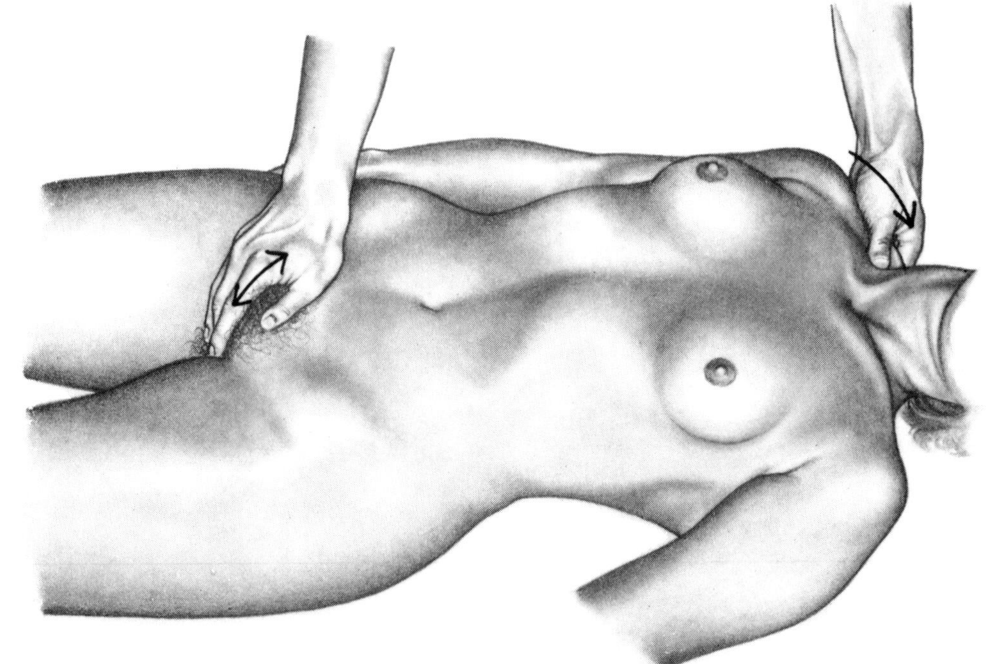

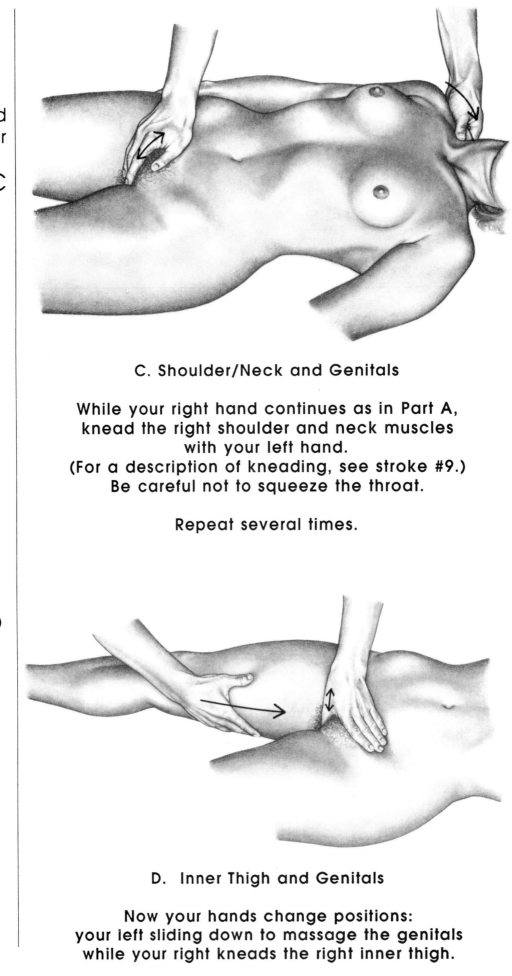

C. Shoulder/Neck and Genitals

While your right hand continues as in Part A,
knead the right shoulder and neck muscles
with your left hand.
(For a description of kneading, see stroke #9.)
Be careful not to squeeze the throat.

Repeat several times.

57. D

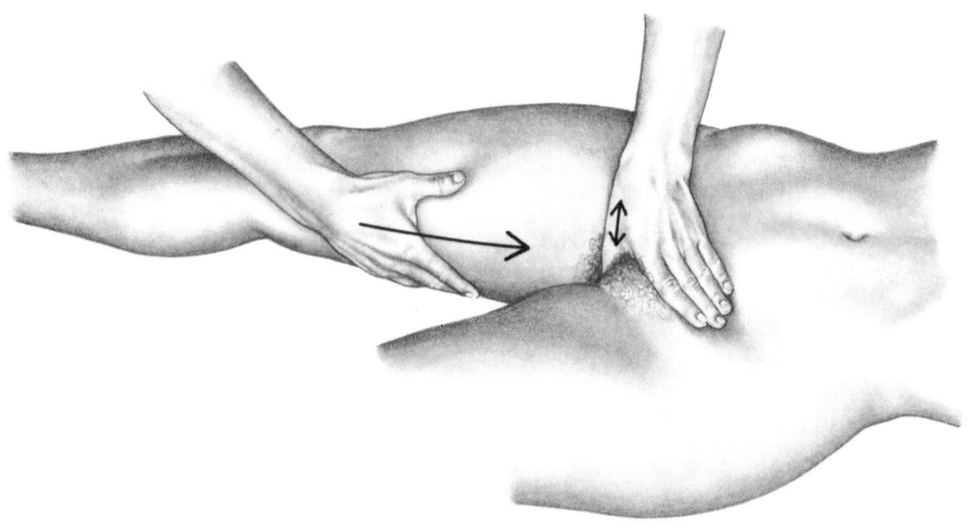

D. Inner Thigh and Genitals

Now your hands change positions:
your left sliding down to massage the genitals
while your right kneads the right inner thigh.

Feelin' Good All Over

57. E

E. Change Sides

If it is possible, move to the other side
and follow the same sequence
while simply reversing
the left-hand and right-hand instructions.
(If you cannot easily move to the over side,
modify your stroking so that the left breast,
neck/shoulder, and thigh areas are massaged also.)

Once you complete this series,
move back to your lover's right side
for the following instructions.
(Remember to keep hand contact if possible.)

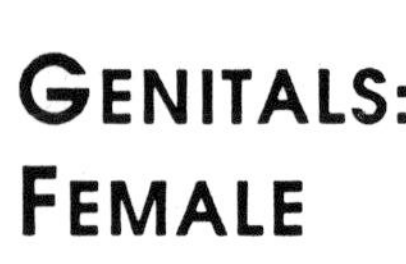


## 58. Being

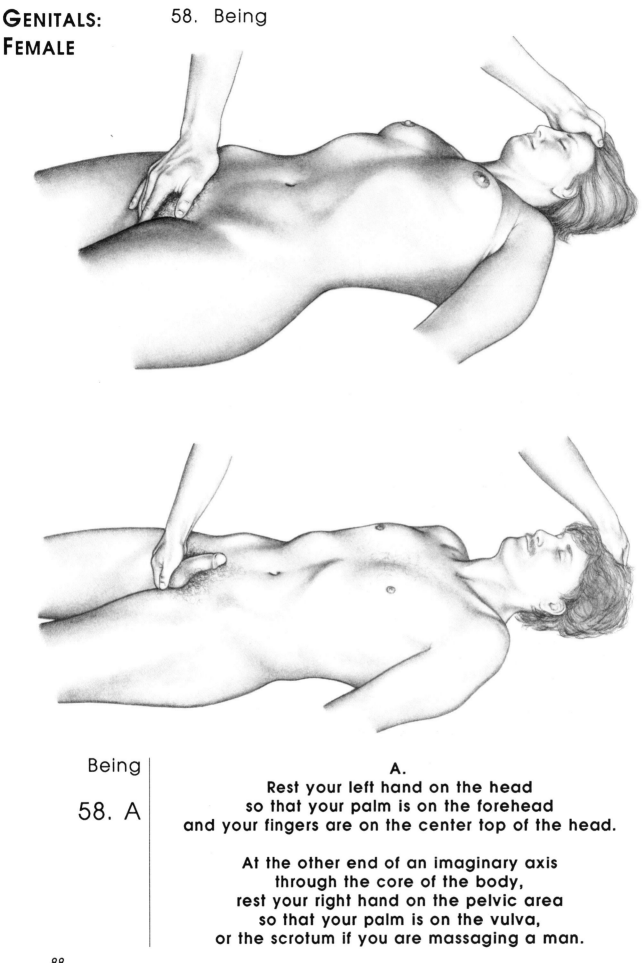

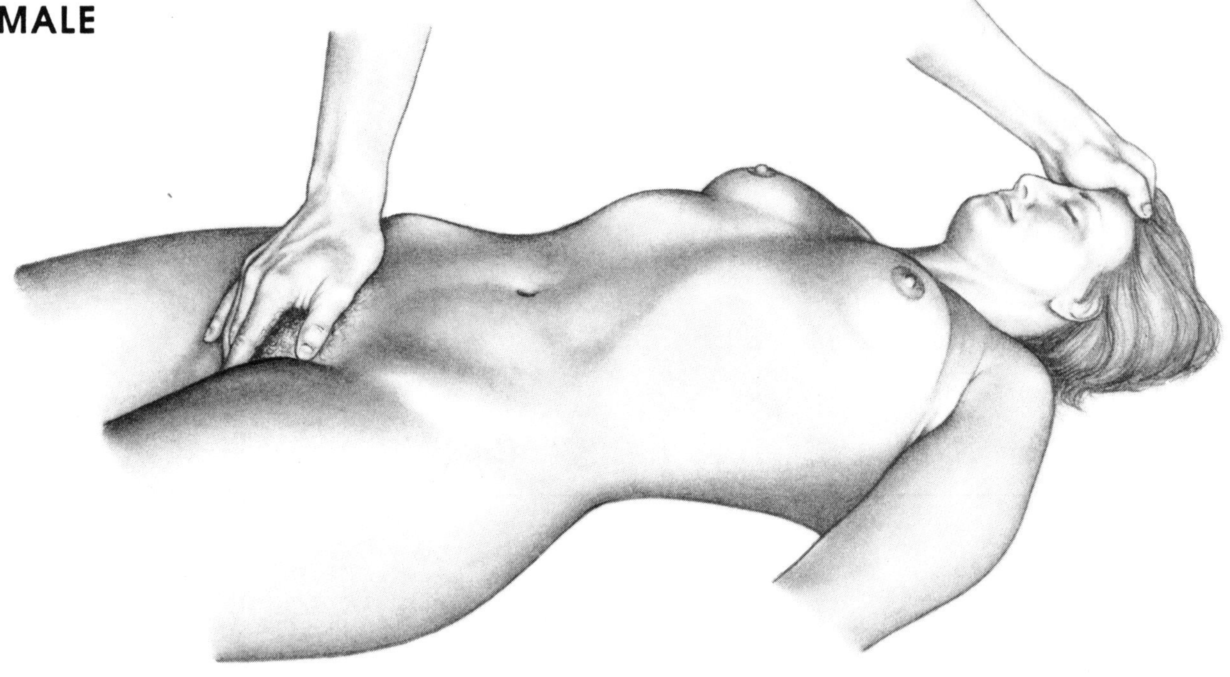

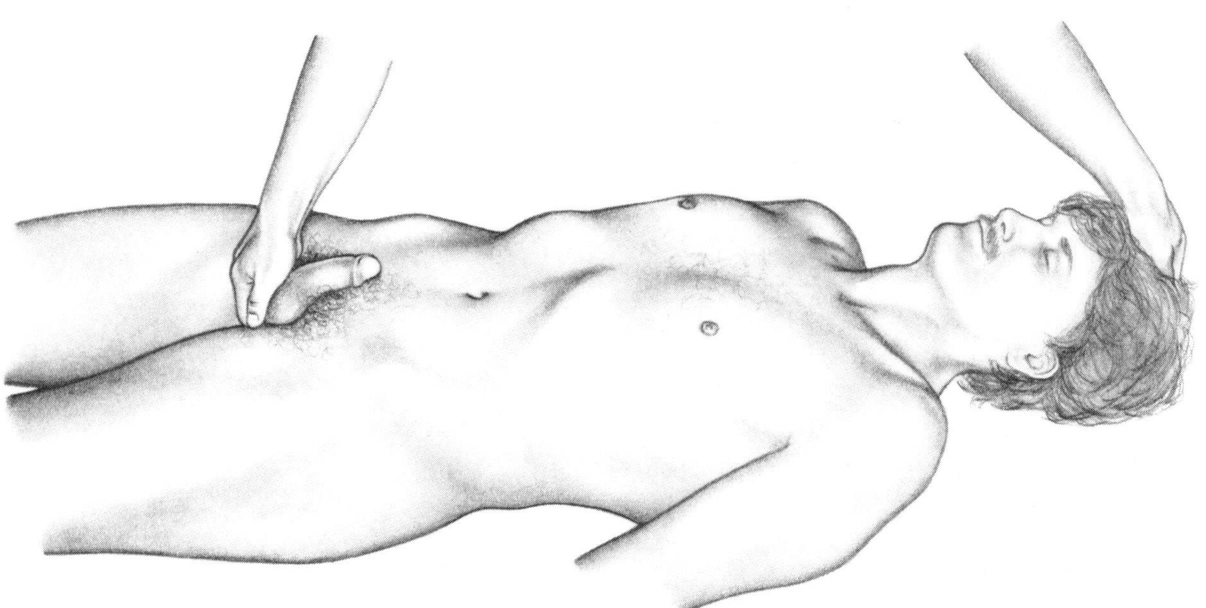

Being

58. A

**A.**

**Rest your left hand on the head**
**so that your palm is on the forehead**
**and your fingers are on the center top of the head.**

**At the other end of an imaginary axis**
**through the core of the body,**
**rest your right hand on the pelvic area**
**so that your palm is on the vulva,**
**or the scrotum if you are massaging a man.**

Being

58. A continued

(58. A continued)

**Now give a soft verbal invitation to your lover
to take a slightly fuller inhalation
and to imagine the breath
beginning at the floor of his/her pelvis
and coming up the core of the body
to the top of his/her head.**

**Then for the exhalation,
invite your lover to simply let go of the breath
and to imagine the breath reversing
and flowing from the top of the head
down through the core of the body
and out the floor of the pelvis.**

**Continue this breathing and imaging guidance
for perhaps two to five minutes.**

Being

58. B

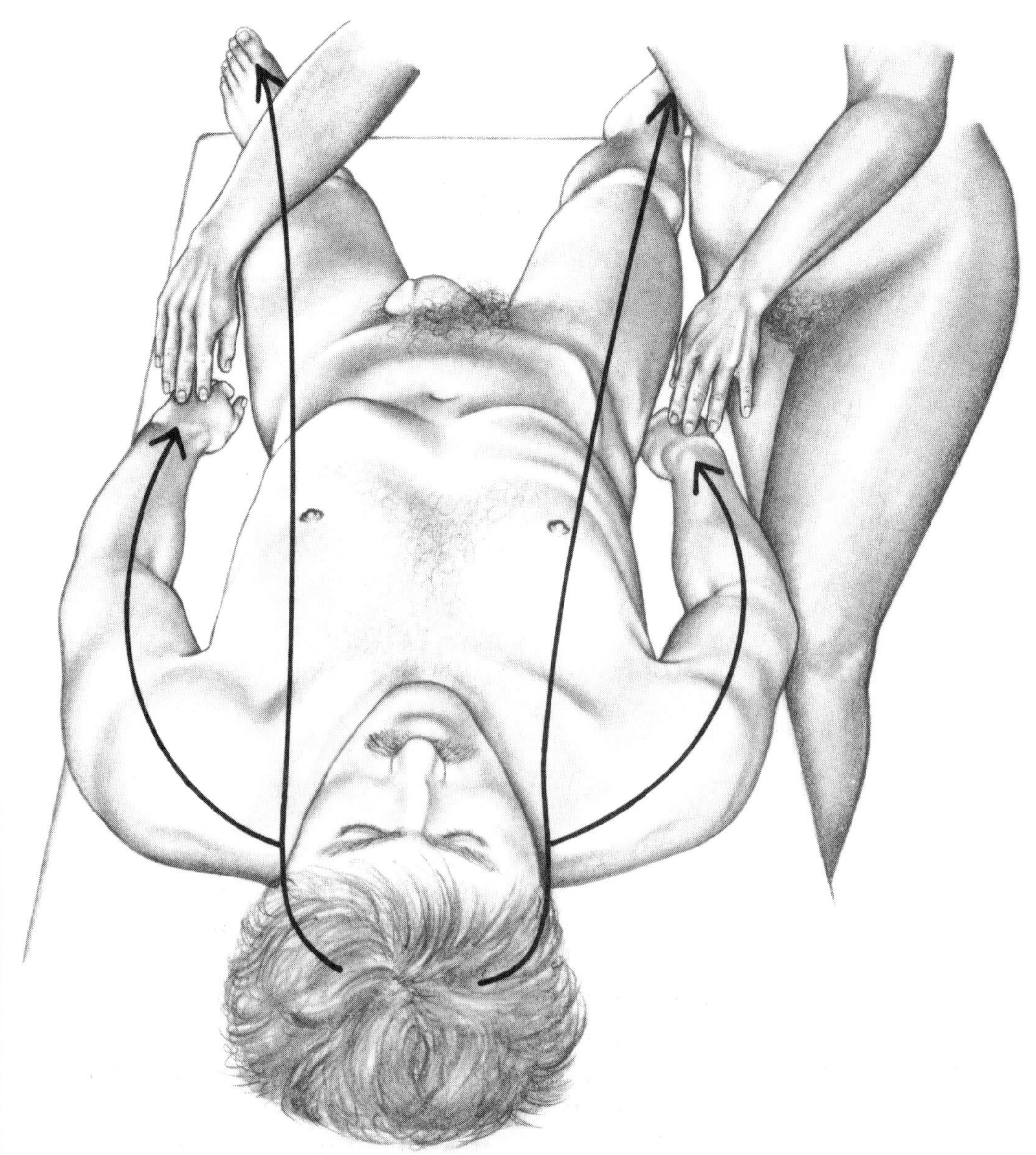

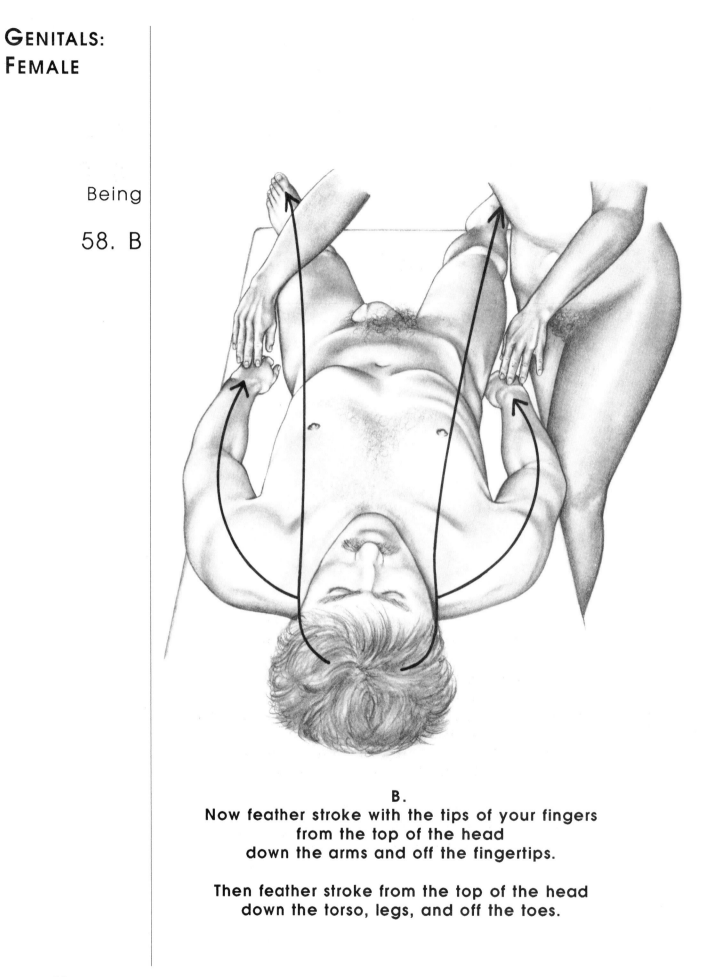

**B.**
**Now feather stroke with the tips of your fingers from the top of the head down the arms and off the fingertips.**

**Then feather stroke from the top of the head down the torso, legs, and off the toes.**

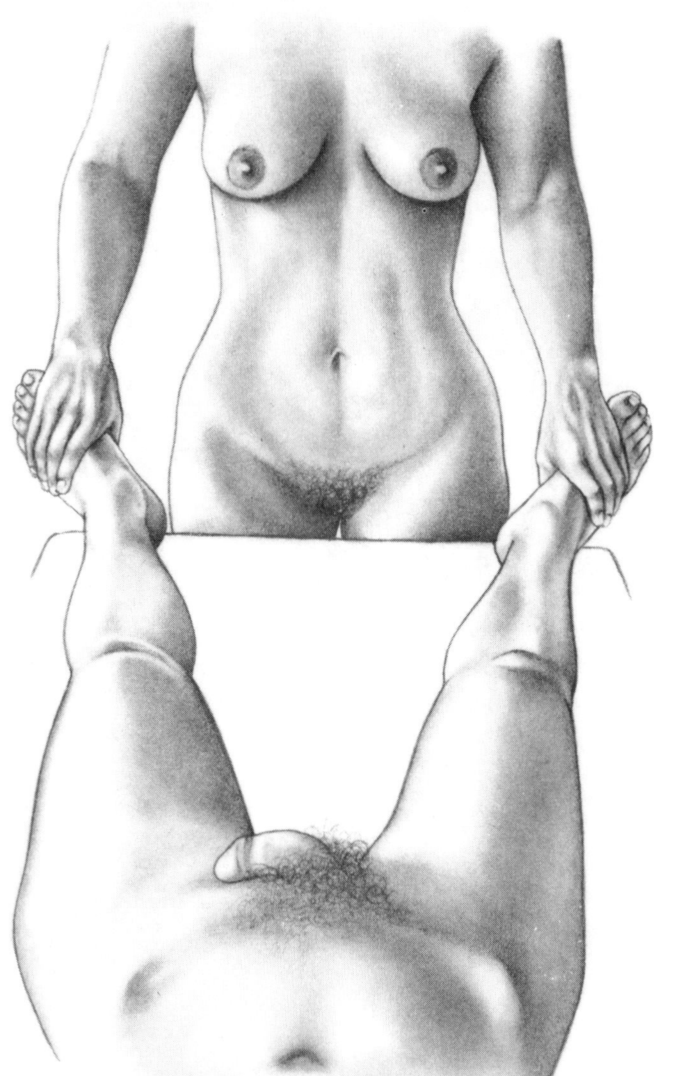

C.

Now rest your hands on the feet
with your thumbs on the arches
and your fingers on top of the feet.

Here again softly give breathing
and imaging instructions:
the inhalation comes from the bottom of the feet
up to the top of the head
The exhalation flows from the top of the head
down to the bottom of the feet.

After a couple of minutes
gradually allow your hands to ascend
up off your lover's feet.

# NECK AND HEAD

Your Position: Behind the head.

## 59. Connecting Stroke

Connecting Stroke

59. A

**A.**
**Place your left hand on the left side of the head so that your thumb is in front of the ear and the fingers are behind the ear.**

**Then rotate the head toward the left shoulder.**

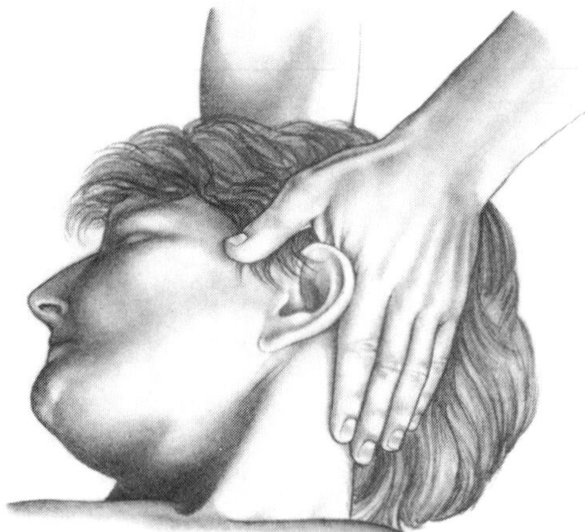

59. B

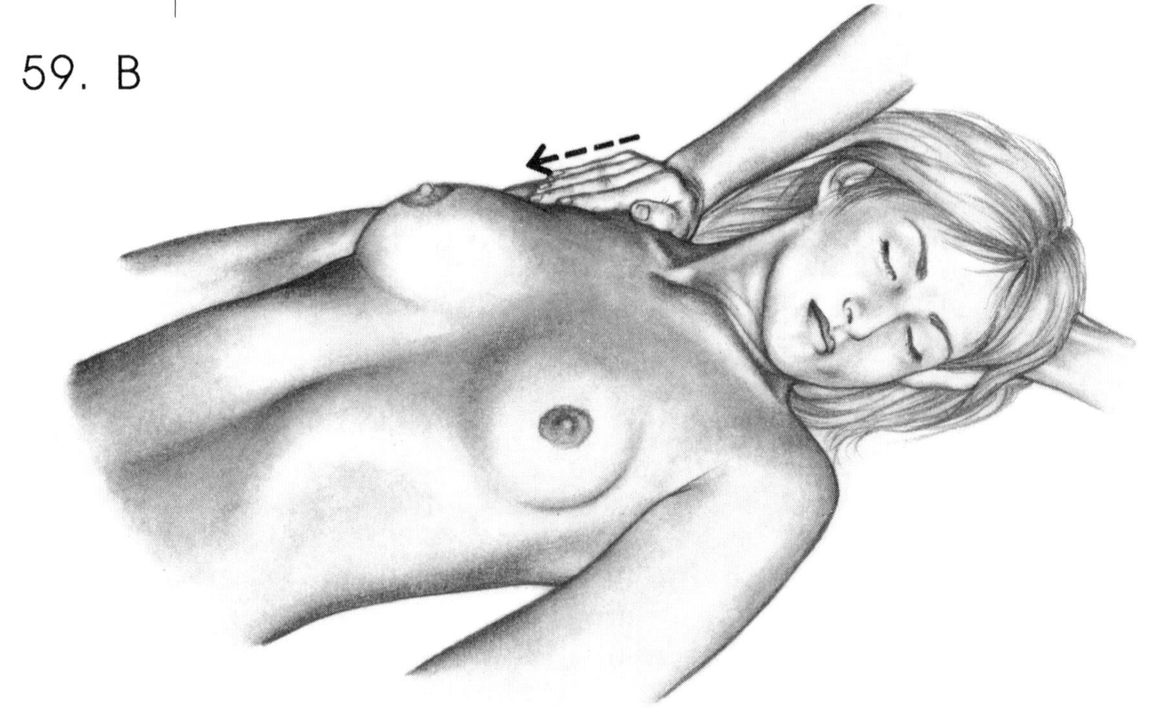

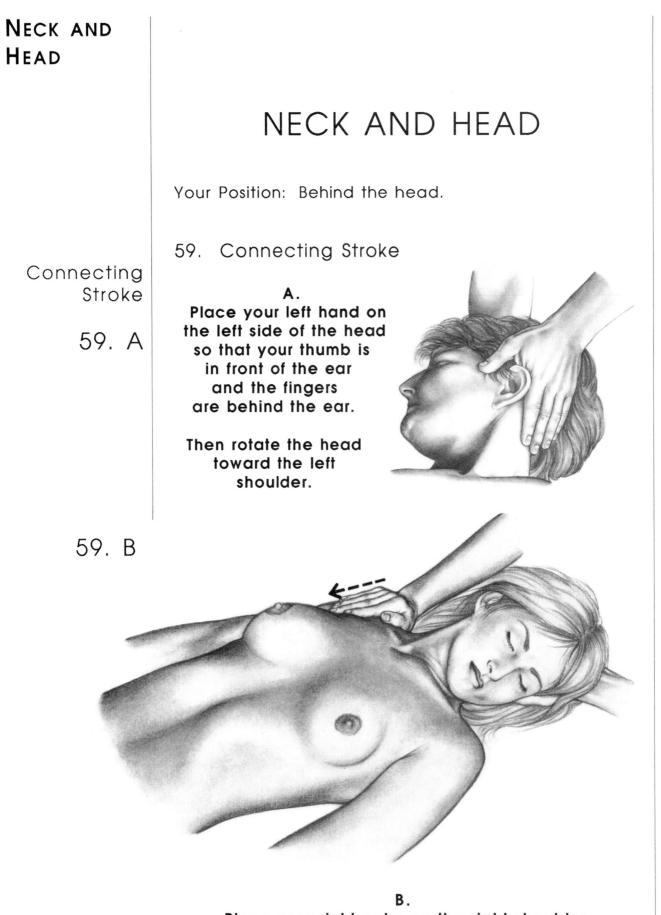

**B.**
**Place your right palm on the right shoulder and stretch downward.**

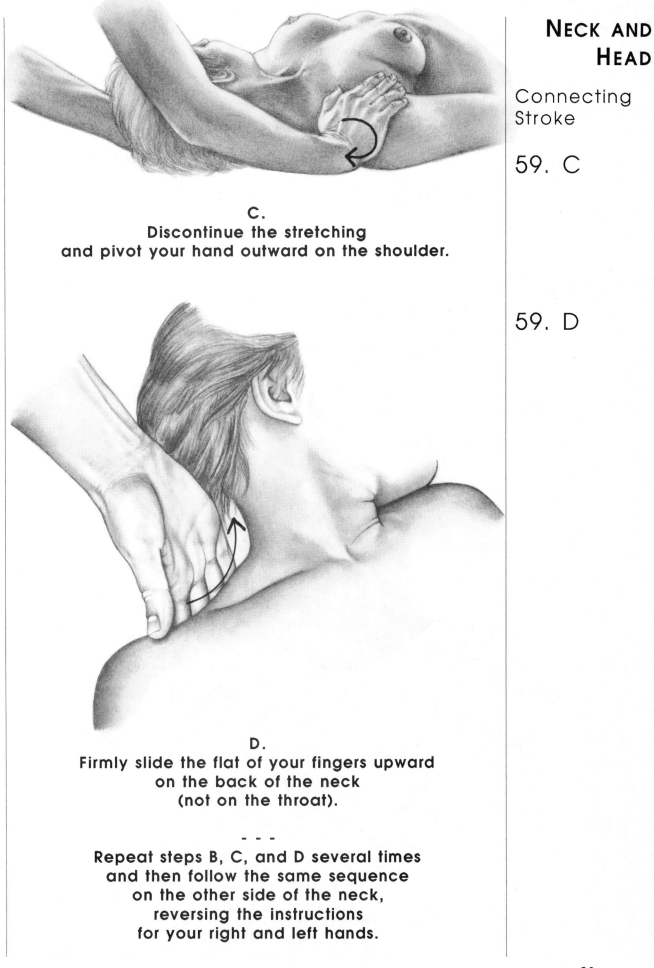

Connecting Stroke

59. C

C.
Discontinue the stretching
and pivot your hand outward on the shoulder.

59. D

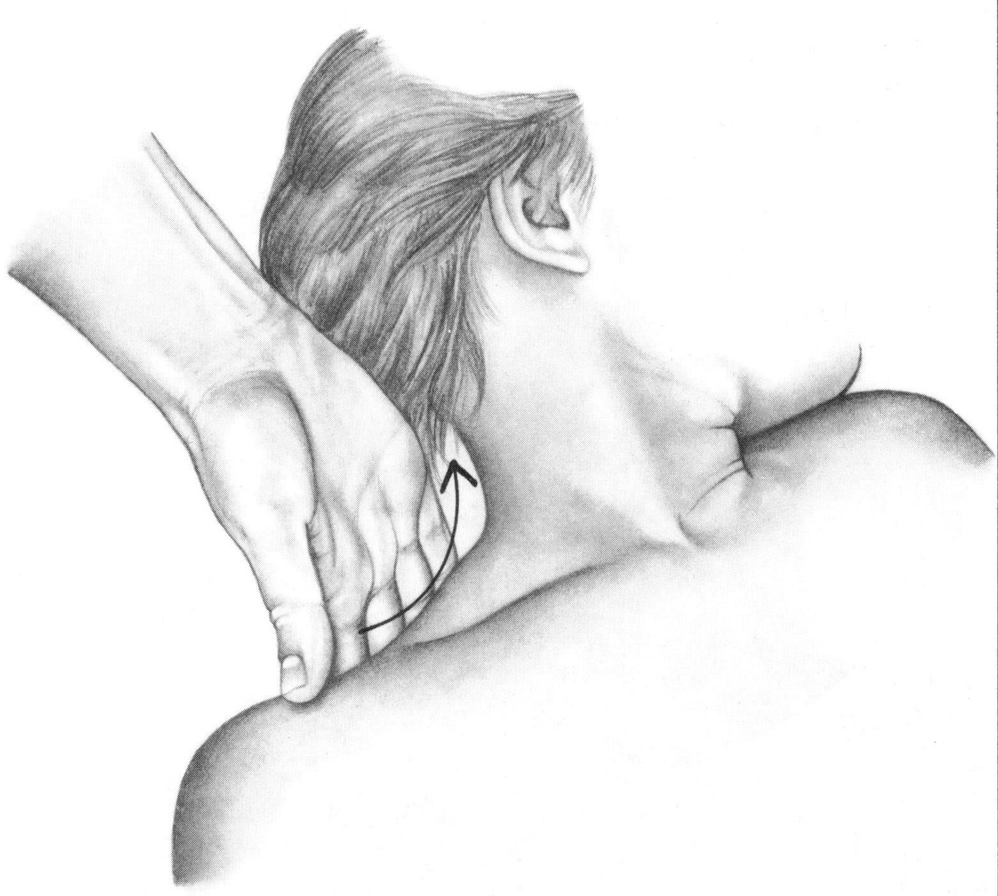

D.
Firmly slide the flat of your fingers upward
on the back of the neck
(not on the throat).

\- - -

Repeat steps B, C, and D several times
and then follow the same sequence
on the other side of the neck,
reversing the instructions
for your right and left hands.

# Neck and Head

Let The Fingers Do The Walking

60.

## 60. Let The Fingers Do The Walking

**With the head resting on the heels of your palms, "walk" the finger pads upward on the back of the neck.**

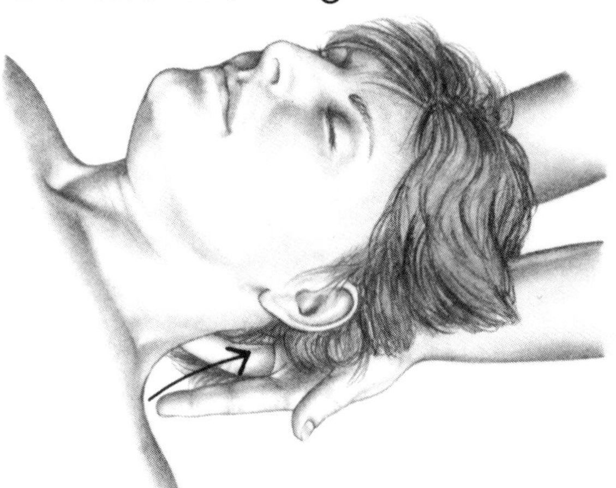

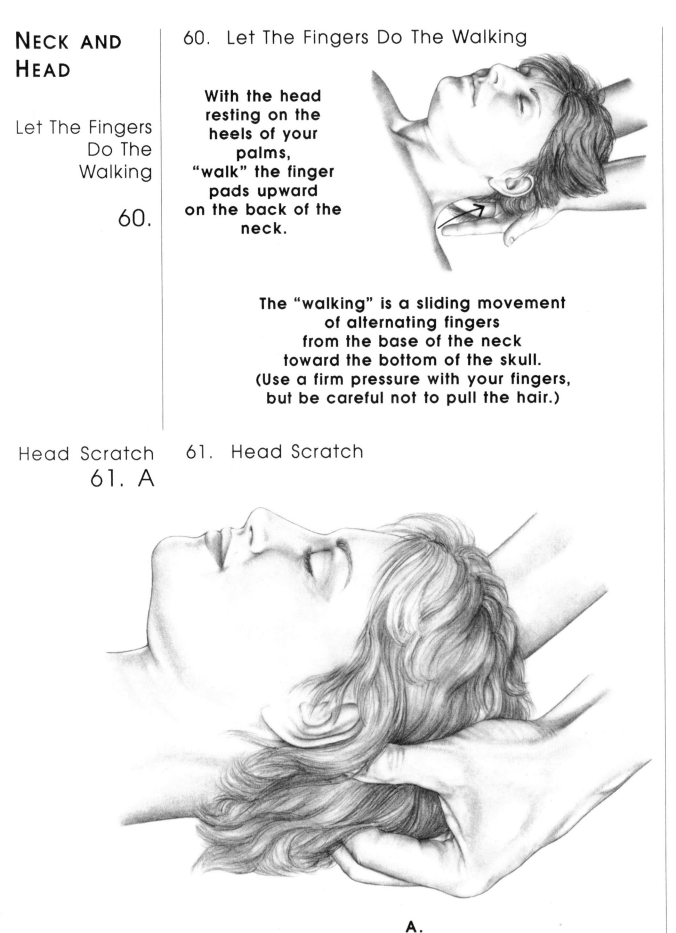

**The "walking" is a sliding movement of alternating fingers from the base of the neck toward the bottom of the skull. (Use a firm pressure with your fingers, but be careful not to pull the hair.)**

Head Scratch

61. A

## 61. Head Scratch

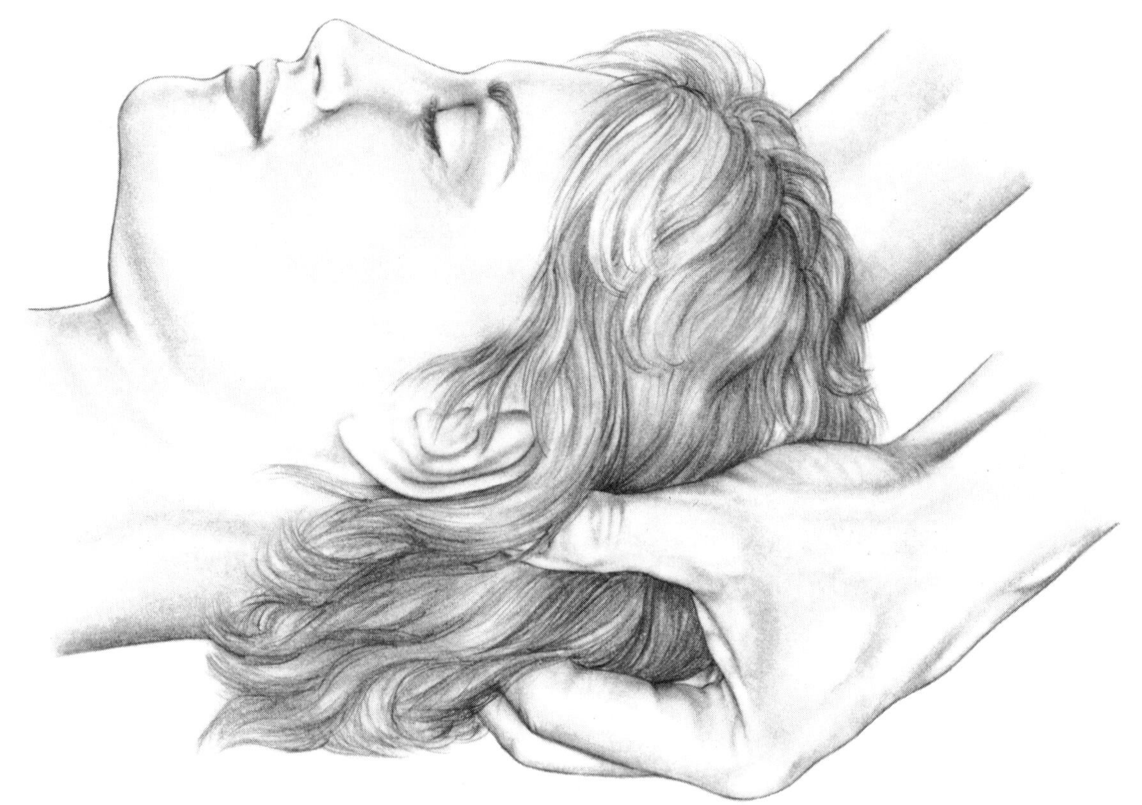

**A.**
**Slide your finger pads back and forth across the scalp on the underneath side of the head.**

## NECK AND HEAD

### Head Scratch

61. B

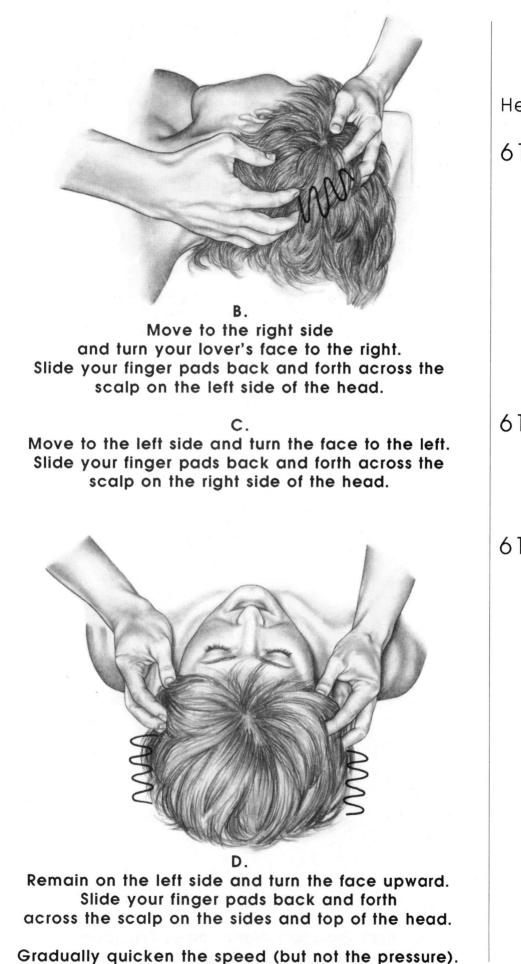

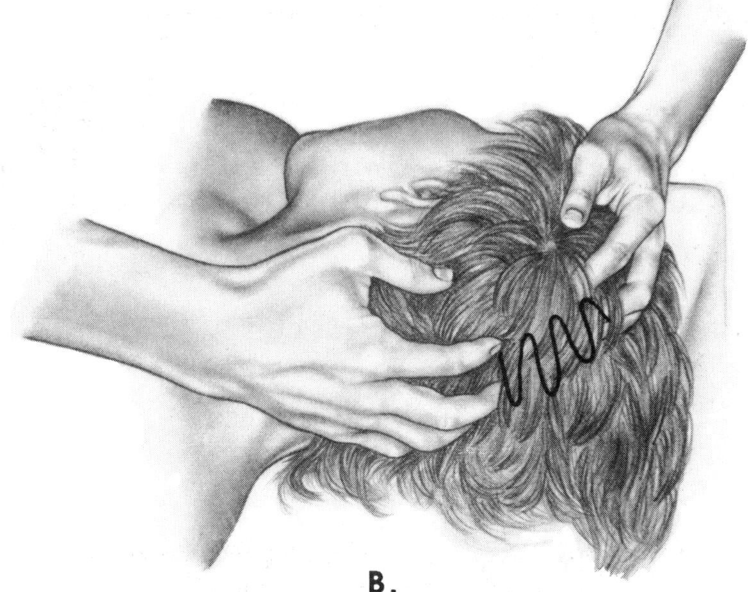

B.
Move to the right side
and turn your lover's face to the right.
Slide your finger pads back and forth across the
scalp on the left side of the head.

61. C

C.
Move to the left side and turn the face to the left.
Slide your finger pads back and forth across the
scalp on the right side of the head.

61. D

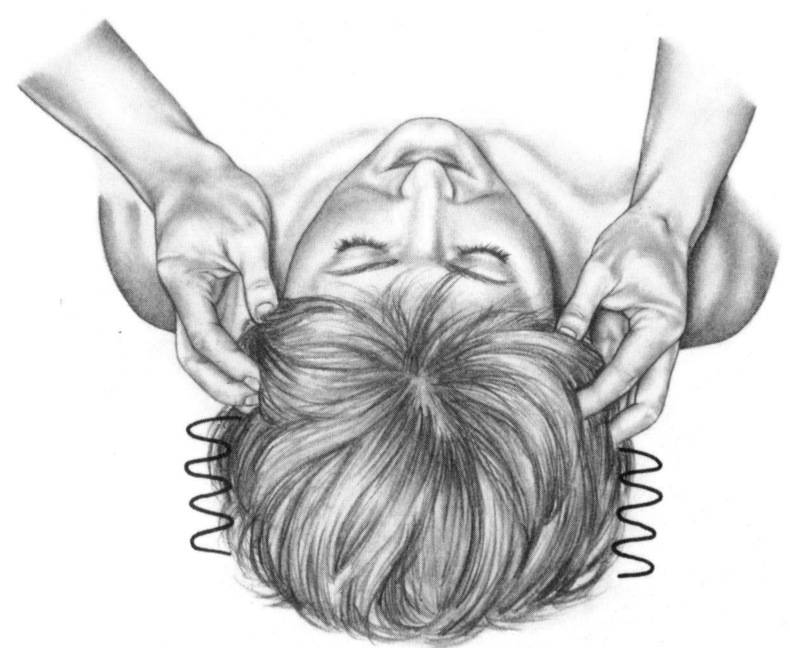

D.
Remain on the left side and turn the face upward.
Slide your finger pads back and forth
across the scalp on the sides and top of the head.

Gradually quicken the speed (but not the pressure).

# NECK AND HEAD

Head Scratch

61. E

E.
**Without slowing down, suddenly lift your fingers off the head.**

61. F

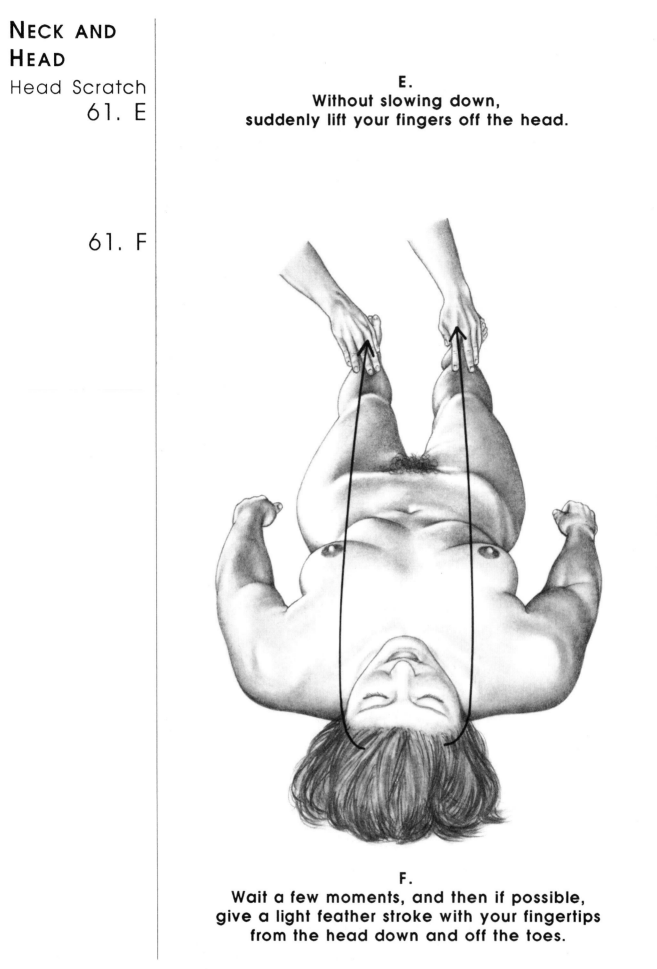

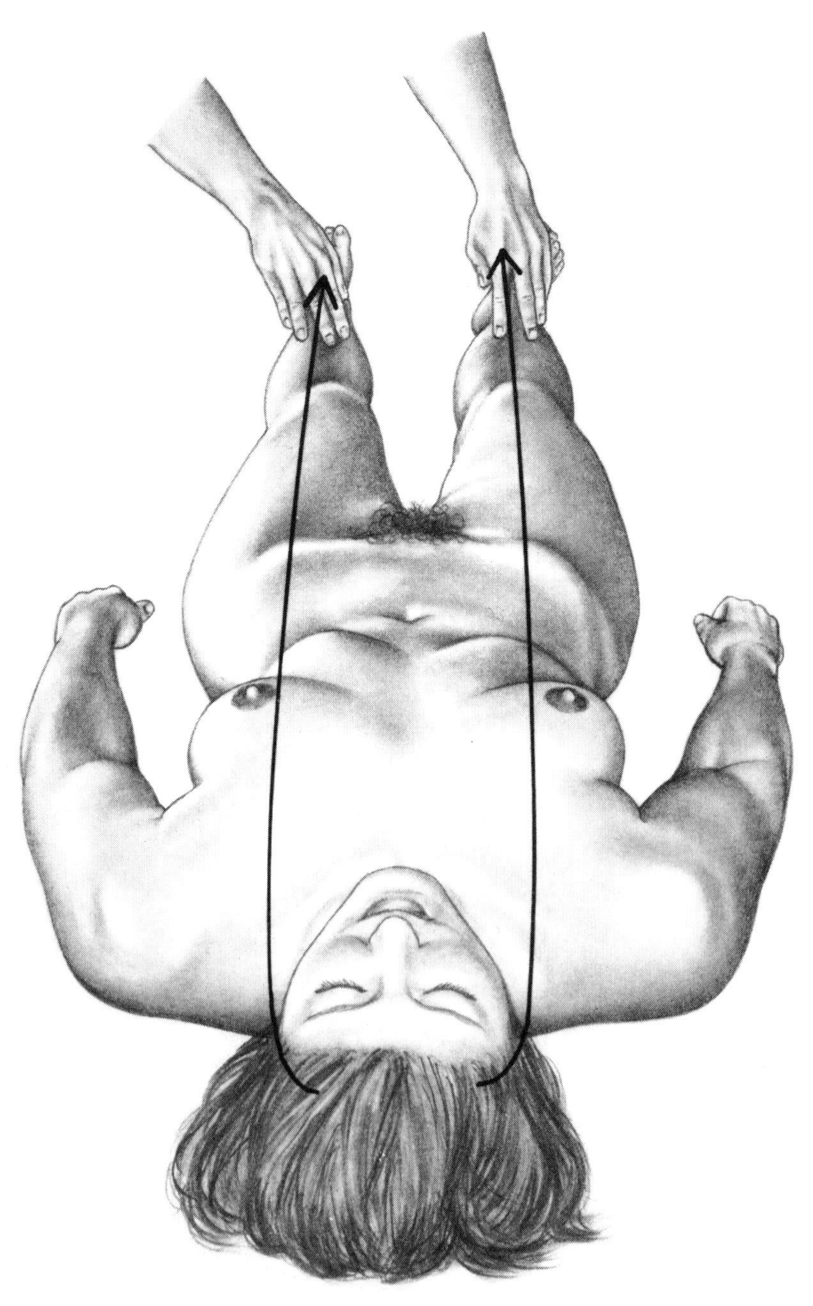

F.
**Wait a few moments, and then if possible, give a light feather stroke with your fingertips from the head down and off the toes.**

# FACE

Your Position: Behind the head.

Note: It is best not to apply more oil for a facial massage. However, if you have been using an unscented oil, you might try a small drop of scented oil.

## 62. T Stroke

T Stroke

62.

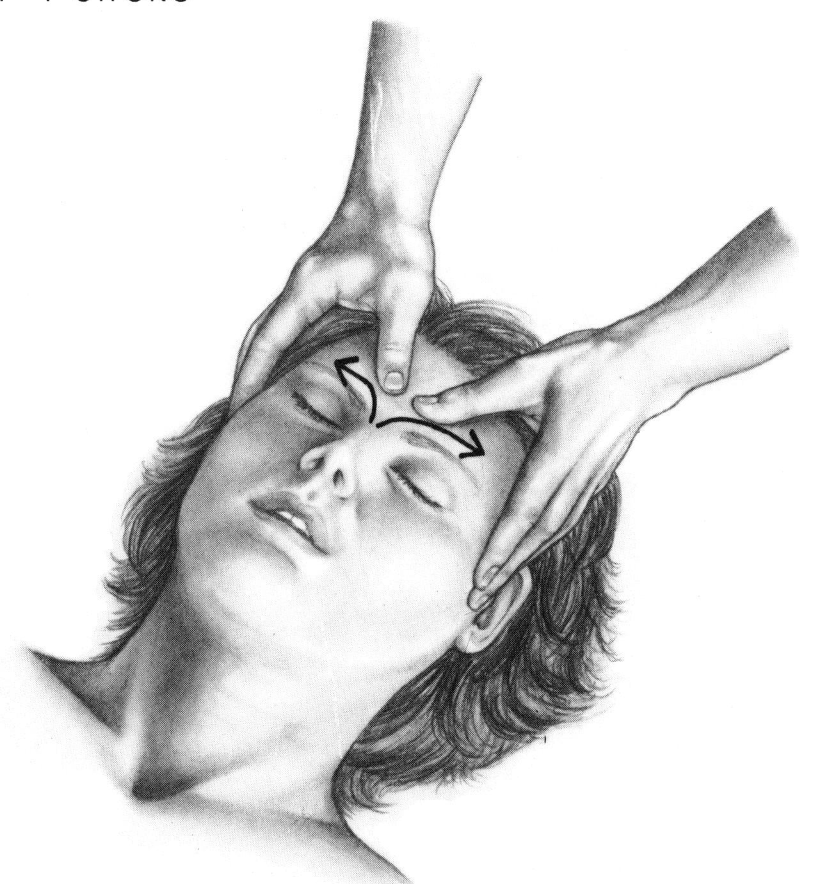

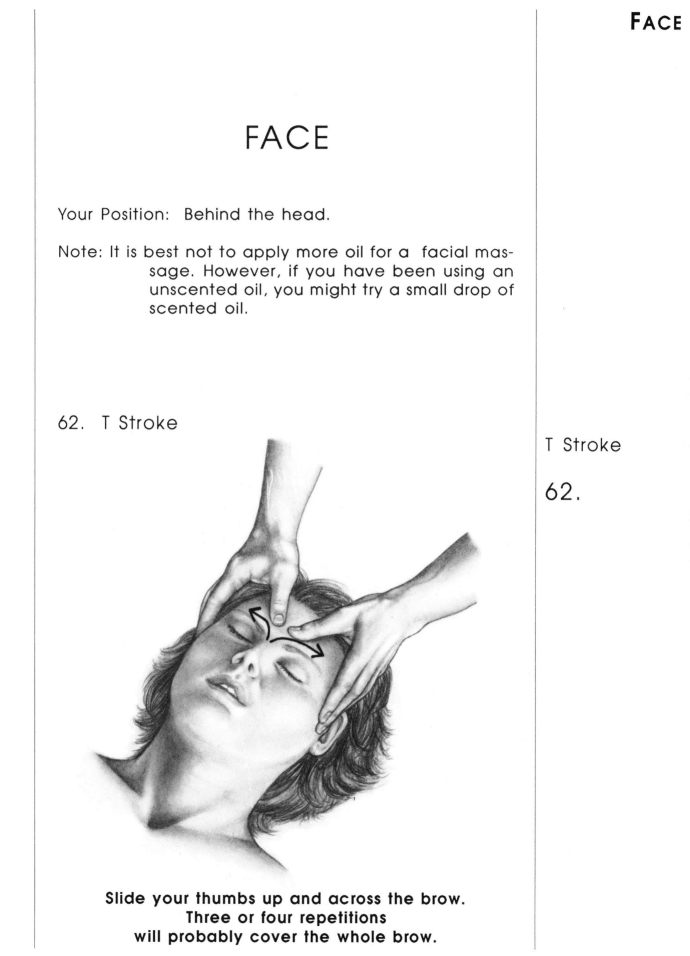

**Slide your thumbs up and across the brow. Three or four repetitions will probably cover the whole brow.**

Eyebrow Squeeze

63.

## 63. Eyebrow Squeeze

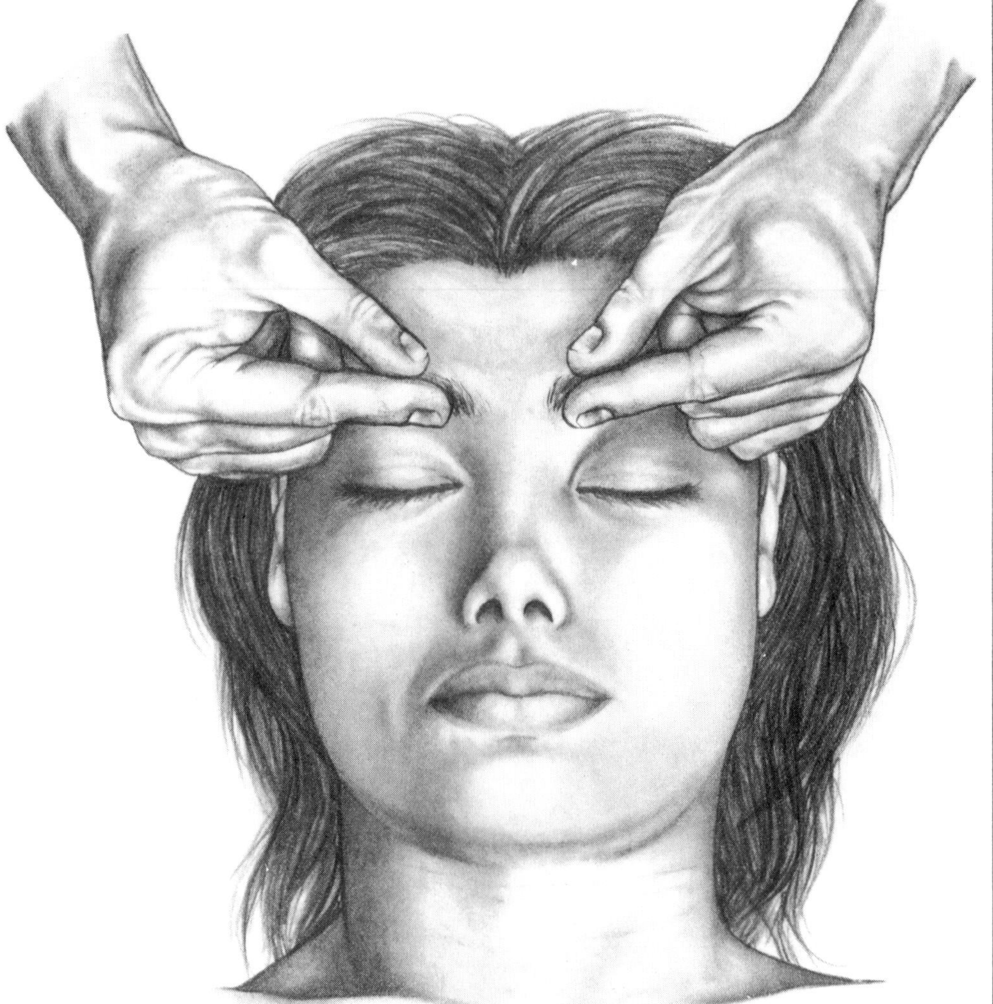

**Make a series of squeezes of the eyebrows from the midline outward.**

## 64. Temple Circles



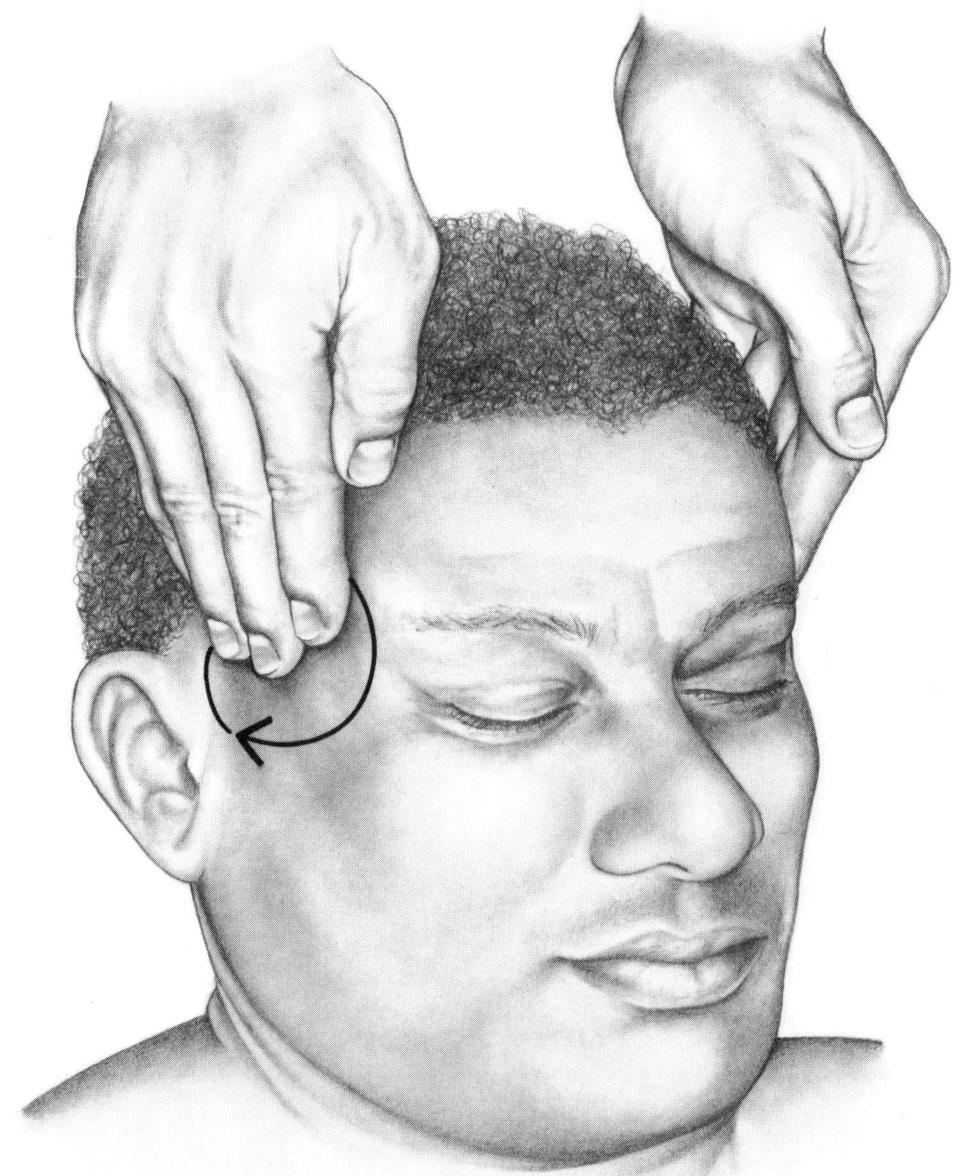

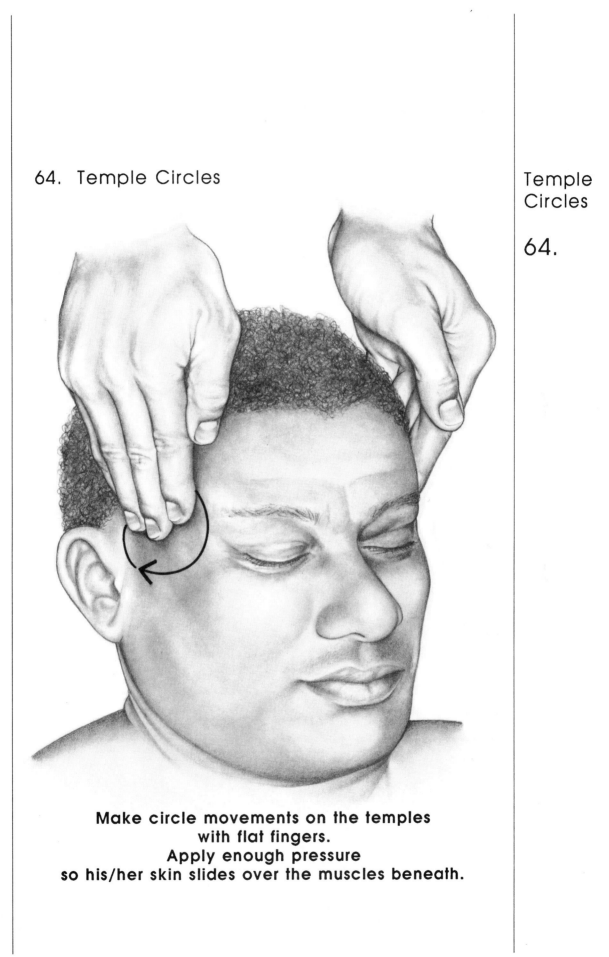

**Make circle movements on the temples with flat fingers. Apply enough pressure so his/her skin slides over the muscles beneath.**

Underneath-The-Eyes Stroke

65.

## 65. Underneath-The-Eyes Stroke

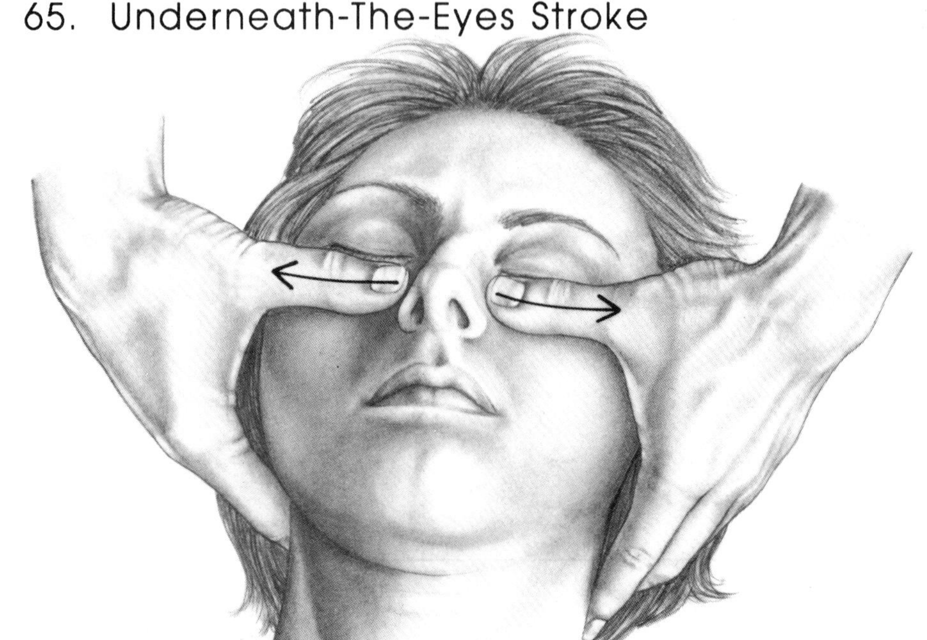

**Slide your thumbs outward across the bony surface underneath the eyes.**

Eye Stroke

66.

## 66. Eye Stroke

**Massage the eyes only if hard contact lens have been removed; light pressure on soft lens may be OK.**

**Bracing the heel of your thumbs on the forehead, slowly slide your thumb pads outward across the closed eyes. Repeat two or three times.**

## 67. Cheek Bone Stroke

Cheek Bone Stroke

67.

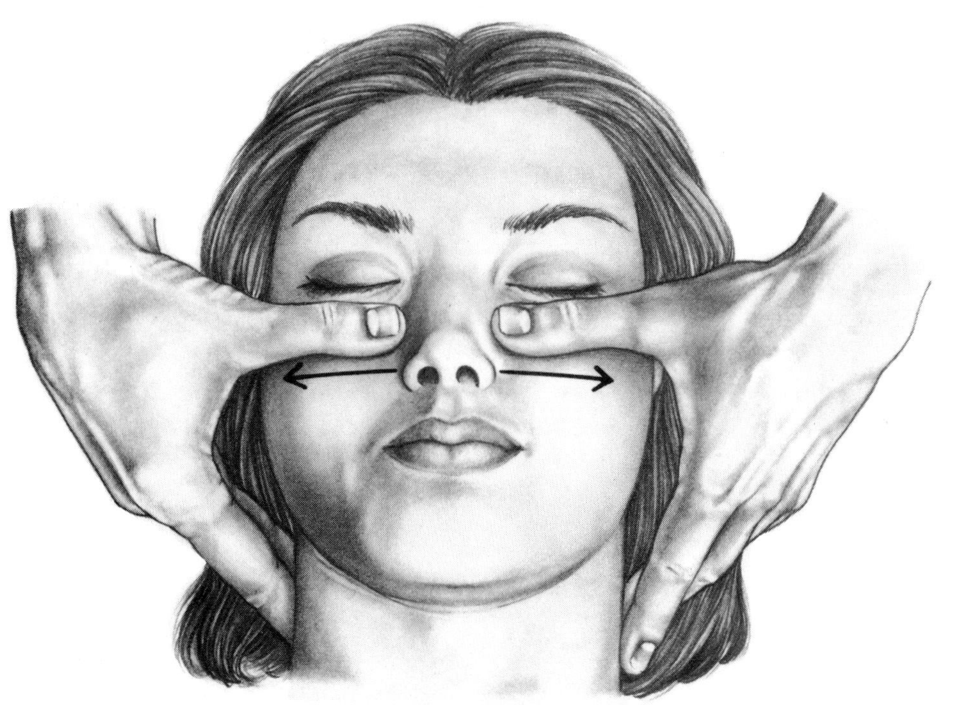

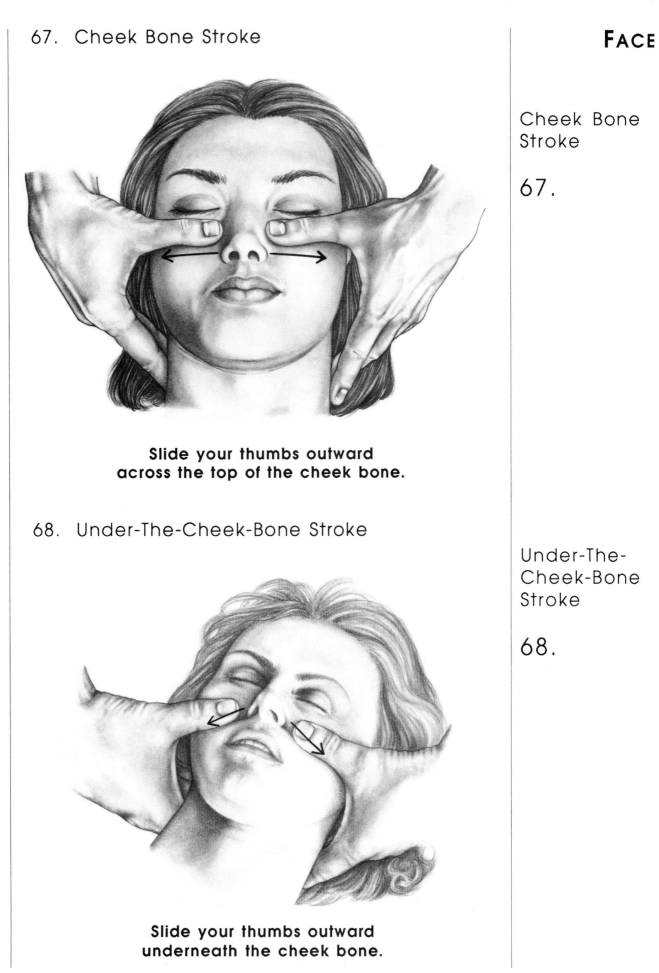

**Slide your thumbs outward across the top of the cheek bone.**

## 68. Under-The-Cheek-Bone Stroke

Under-The-Cheek-Bone Stroke

68.

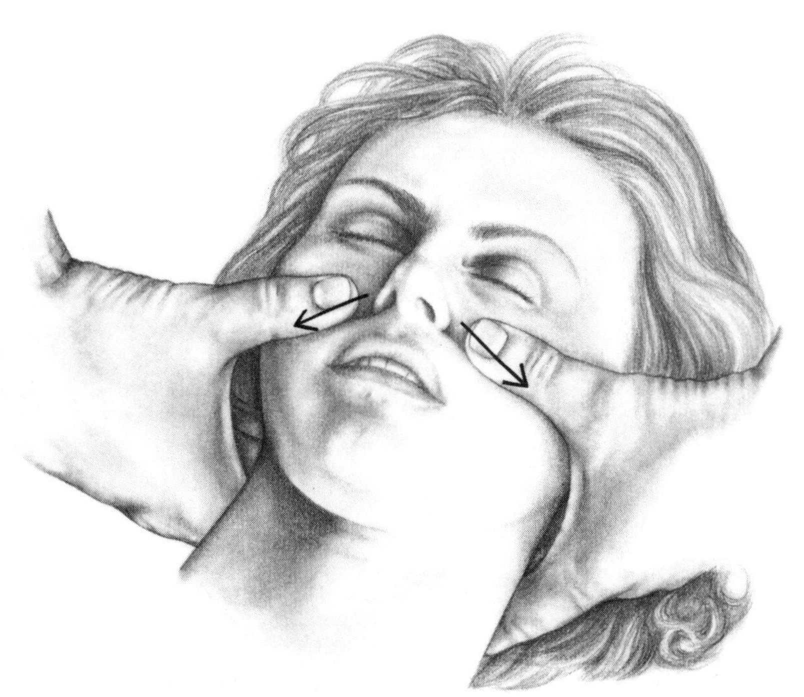

**Slide your thumbs outward underneath the cheek bone.**

Jaw Circles

69.

69. Jaw Circles

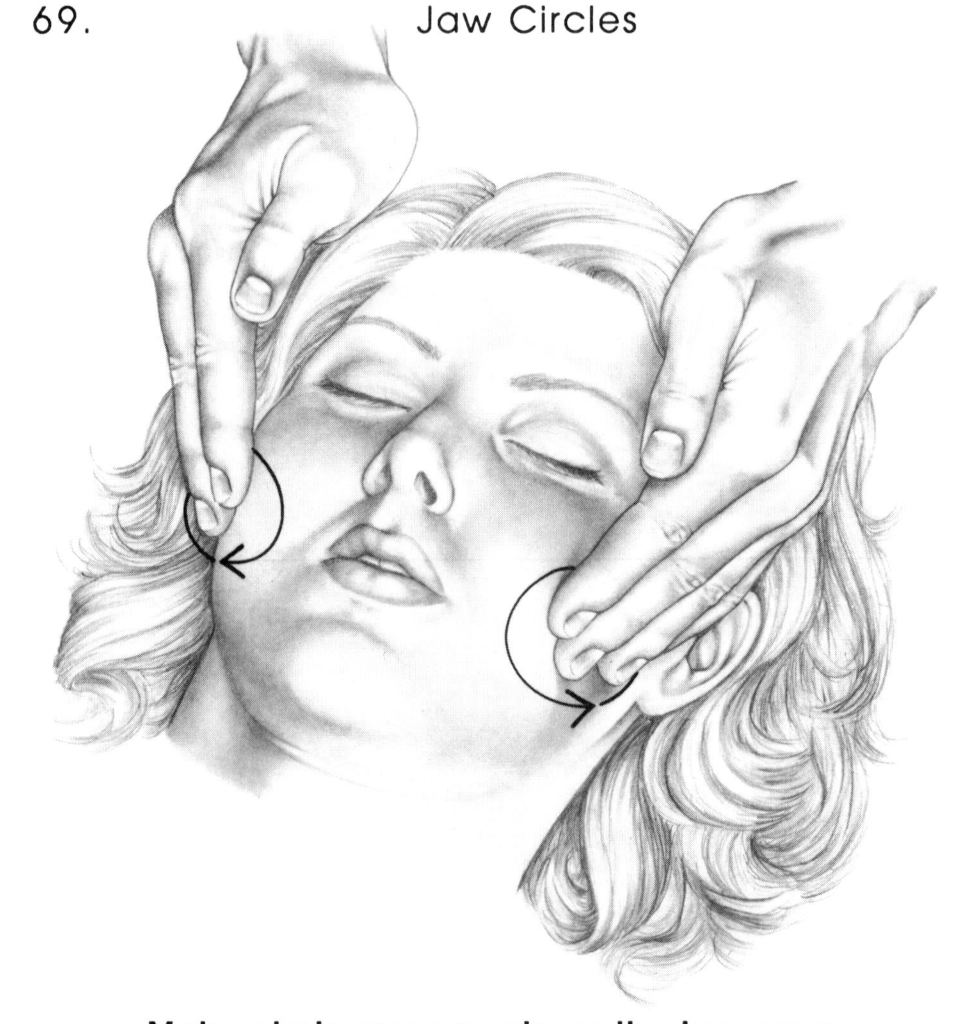

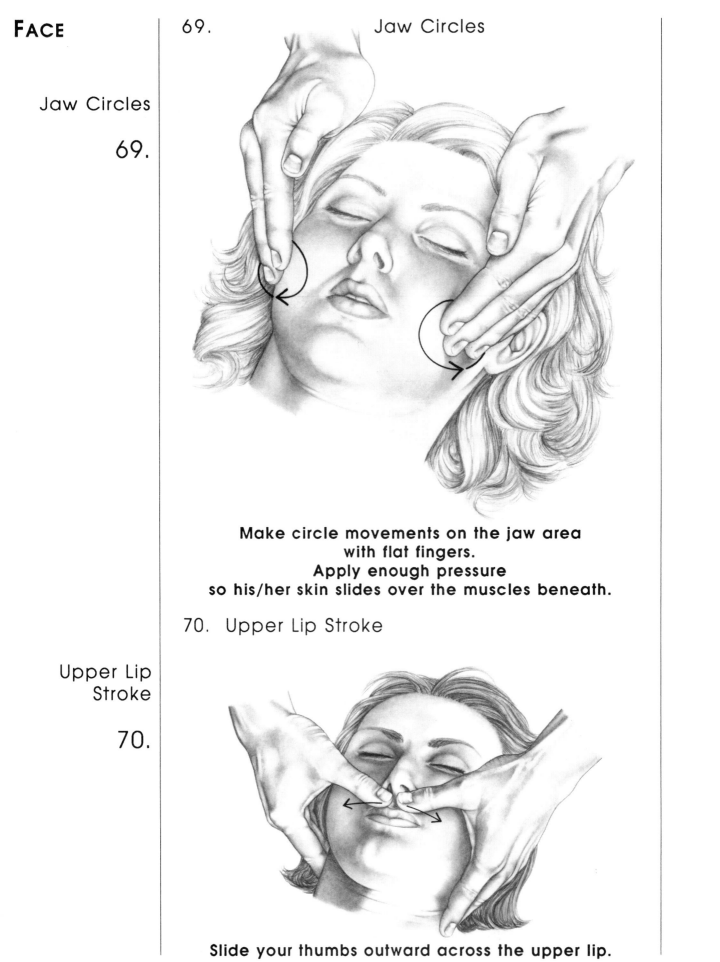

**Make circle movements on the jaw area with flat fingers. Apply enough pressure so his/her skin slides over the muscles beneath.**

Upper Lip Stroke

70.

70. Upper Lip Stroke

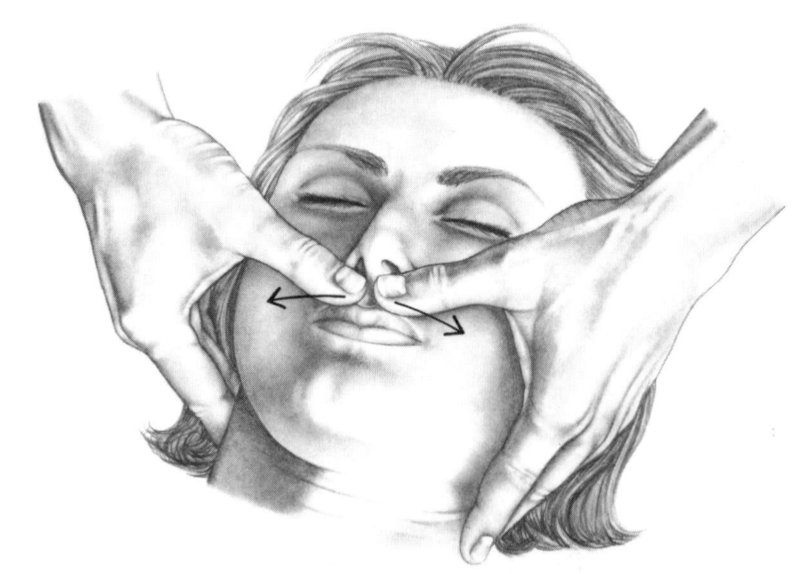

**Slide your thumbs outward across the upper lip.**

## 71. Lower Lip Stroke

Lower Lip Stroke

71.

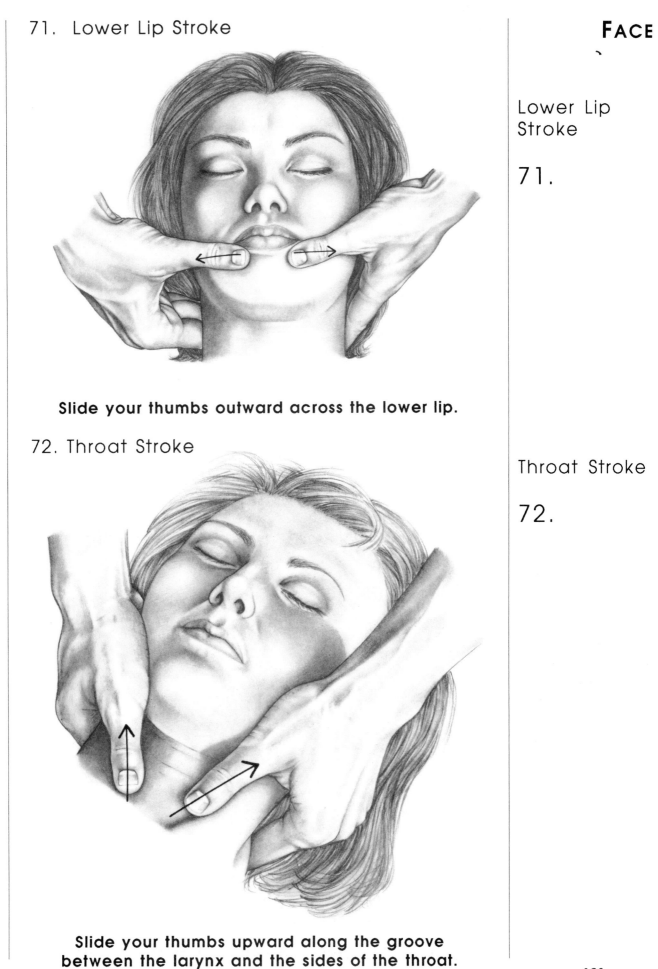

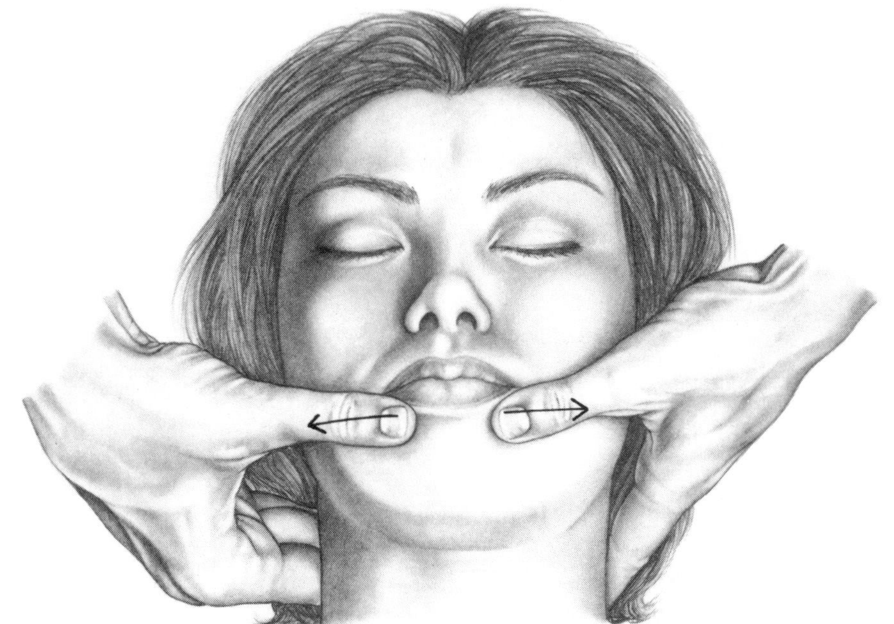

**Slide your thumbs outward across the lower lip.**

## 72. Throat Stroke

Throat Stroke

72.

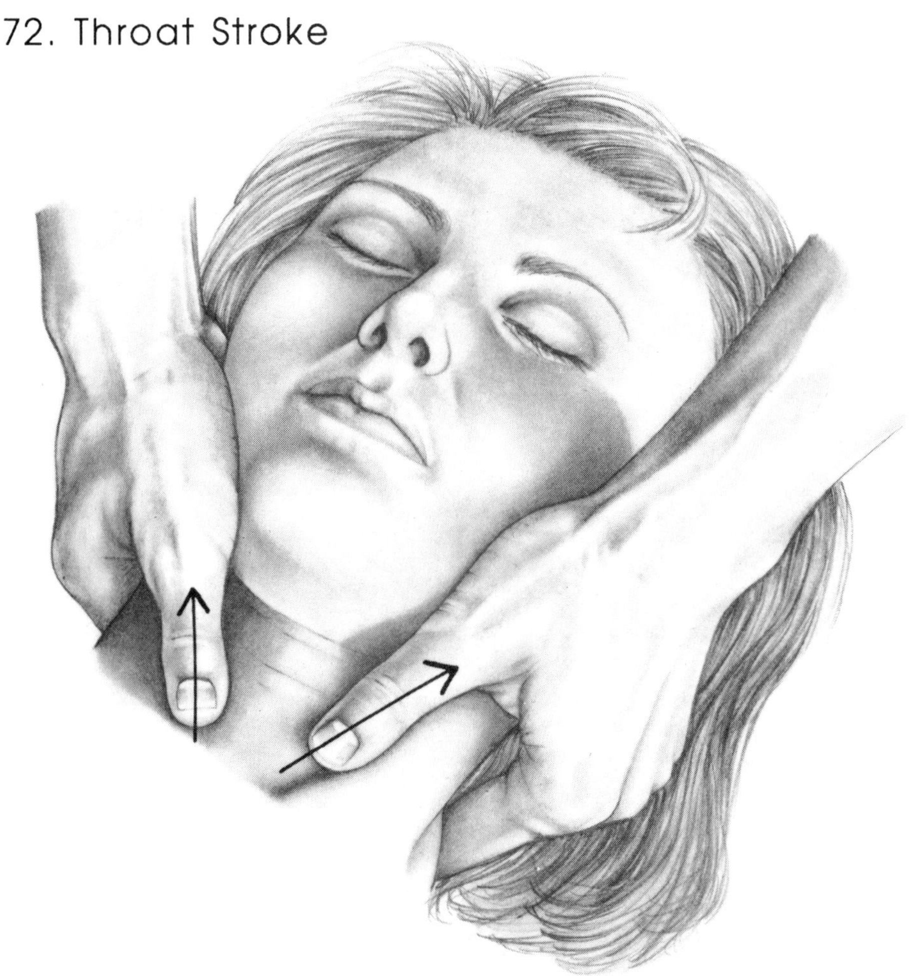

**Slide your thumbs upward along the groove between the larynx and the sides of the throat.**

Behind-The-Ear Stroke

73.

## 73. Behind-The-Ear Stroke

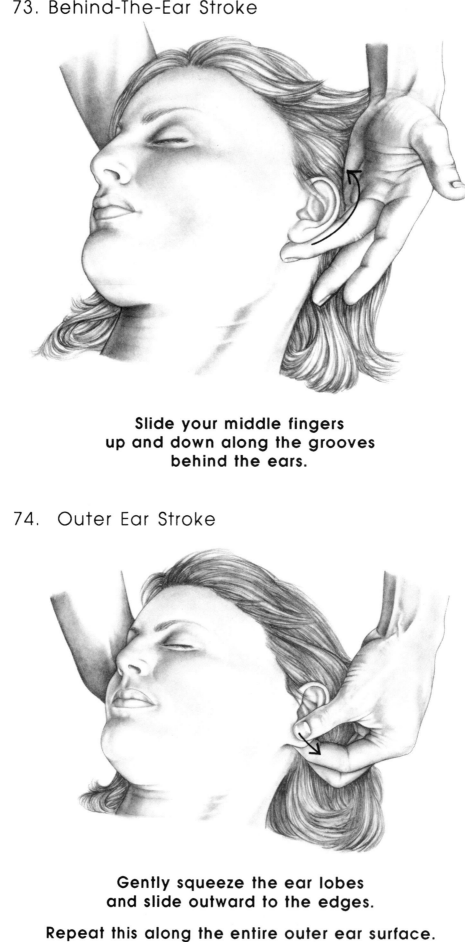

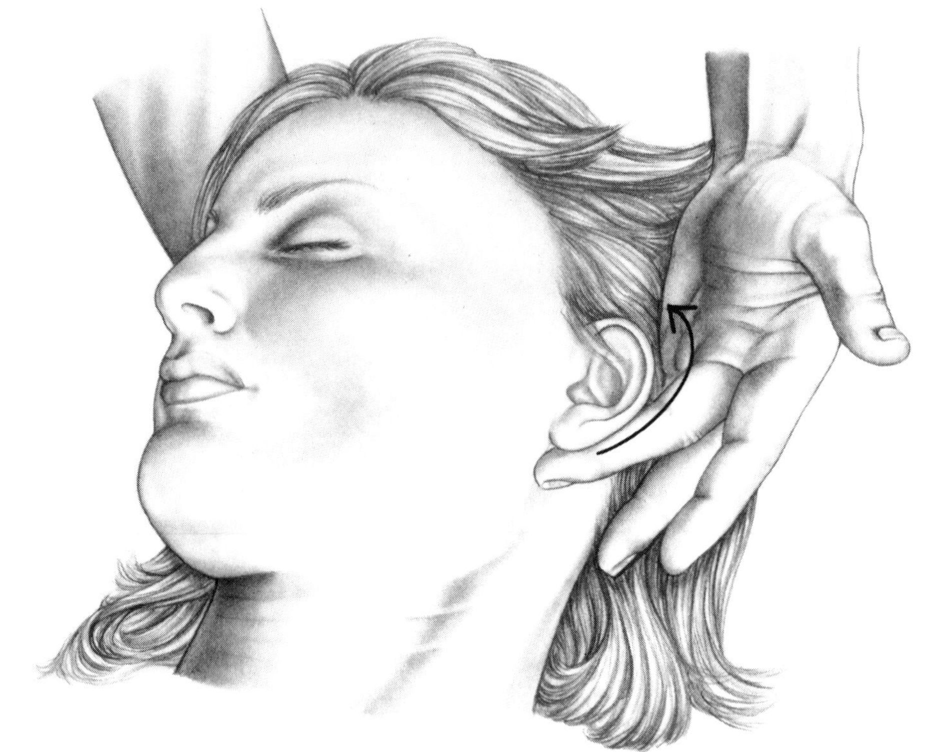

**Slide your middle fingers up and down along the grooves behind the ears.**

Outer Ear Stroke

74.

## 74. Outer Ear Stroke

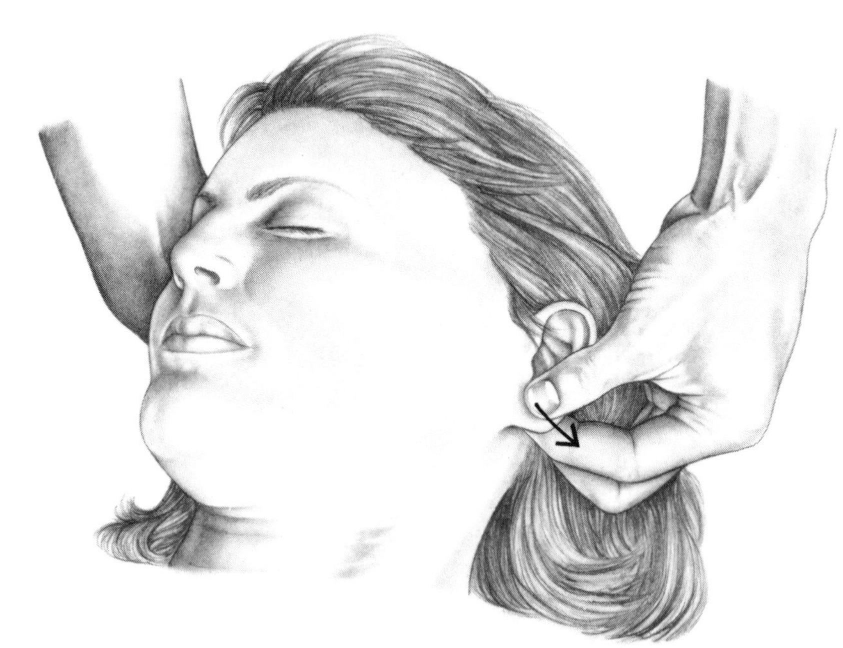

**Gently squeeze the ear lobes and slide outward to the edges.**

**Repeat this along the entire outer ear surface.**

## 75. Inner Peace

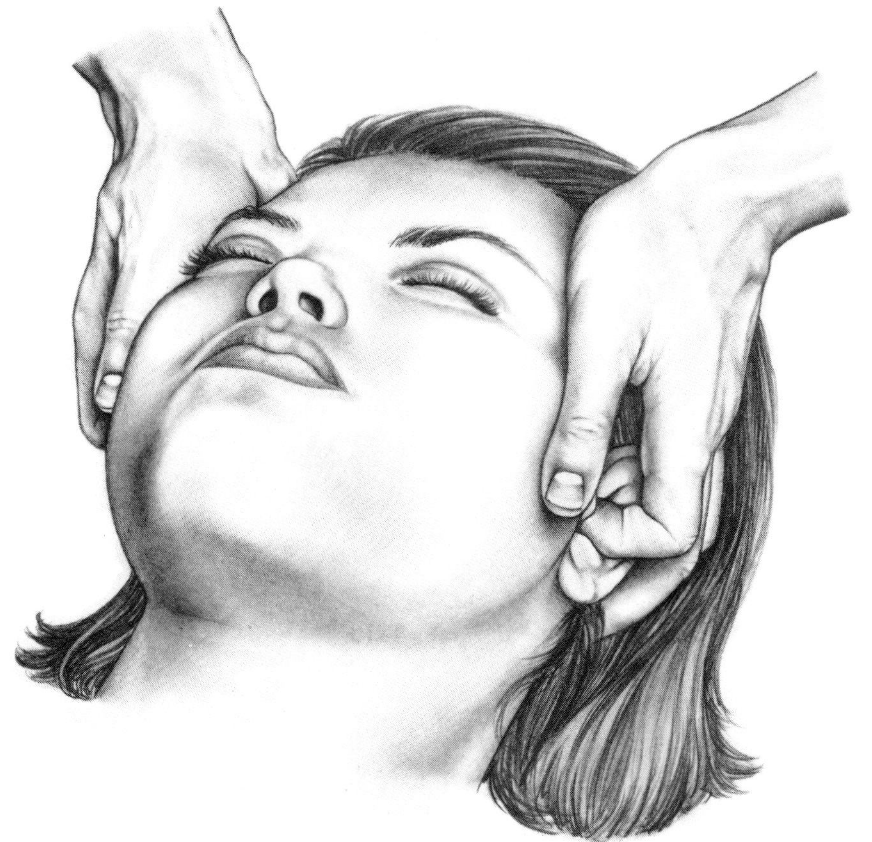

**A.**
**Slowly slide your fingers into the ear canals and relax in this position for about a minute, blocking out the external sounds.**

**B.**
**If Part A is difficult for you or uncomfortable for your lover, cover the ears with your cupped palms.**

Inner Peace

75. A

75. B

# CONCLUSION

## 76. Concluding Stroke

Concluding Stroke

76.

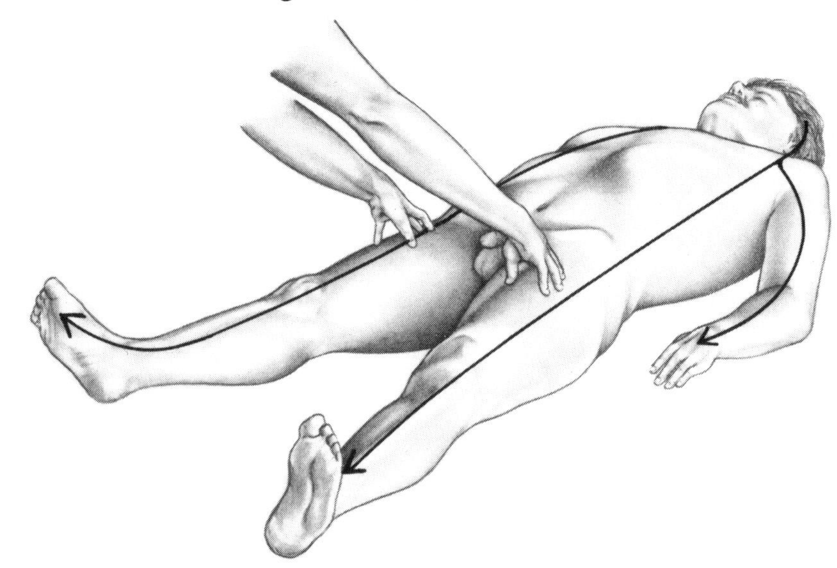

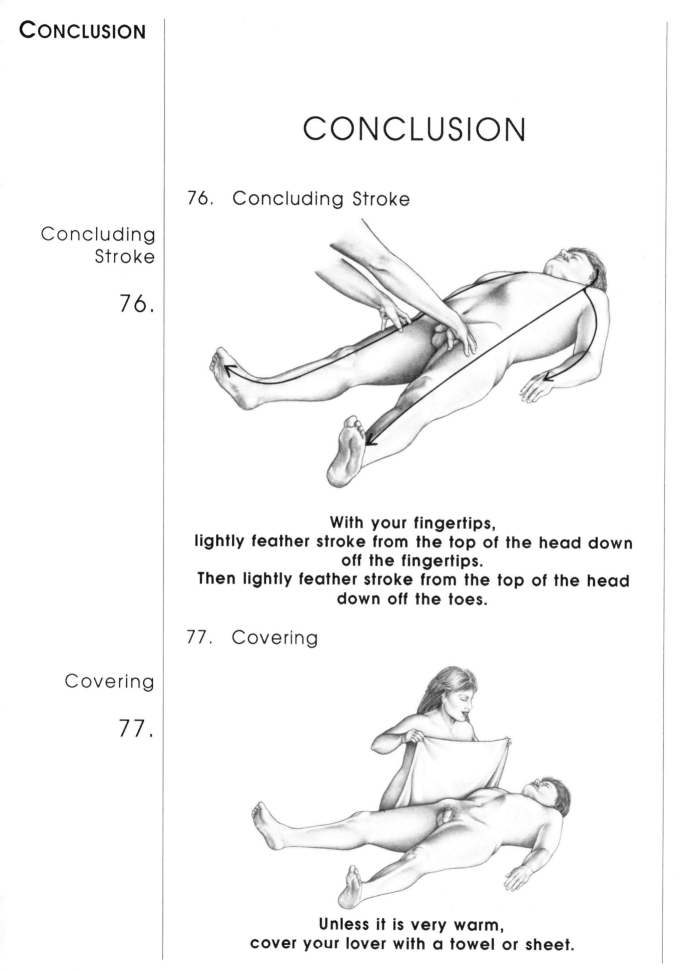

**With your fingertips,
lightly feather stroke from the top of the head down off the fingertips.
Then lightly feather stroke from the top of the head down off the toes.**

## 77. Covering

Covering

77.

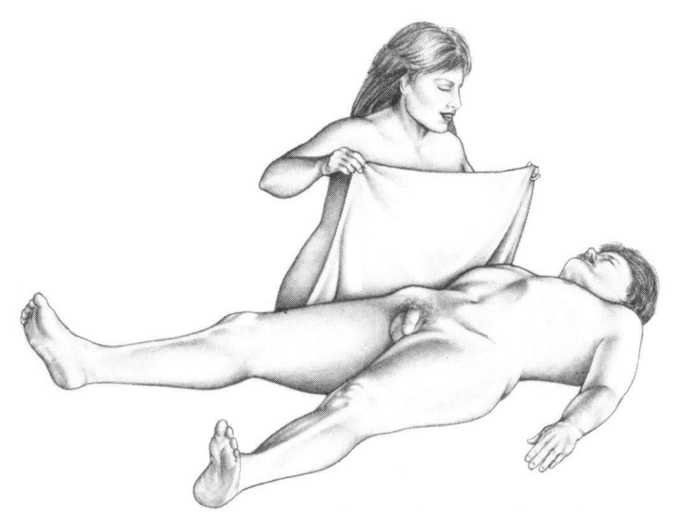

**Unless it is very warm,
cover your lover with a towel or sheet.**

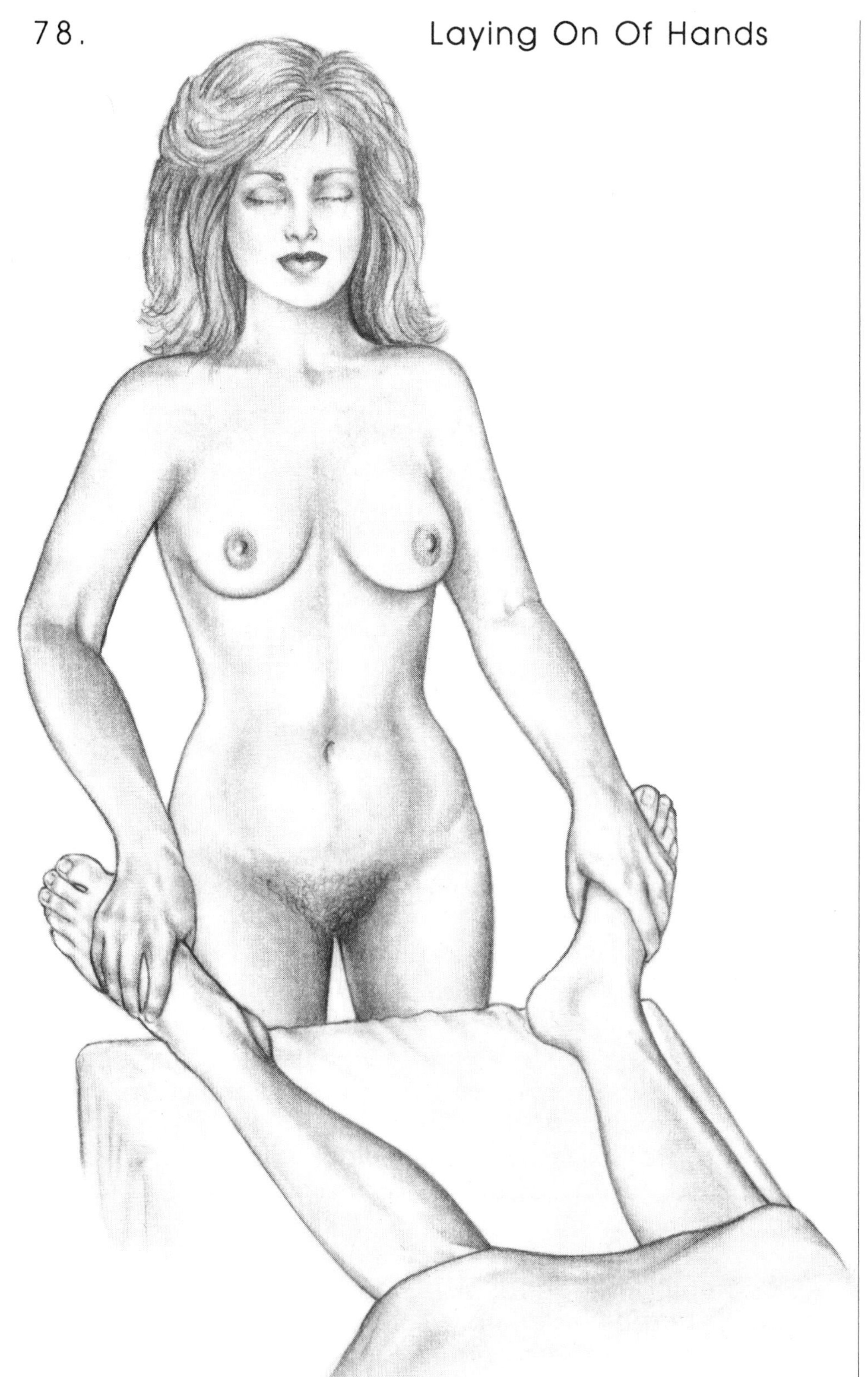

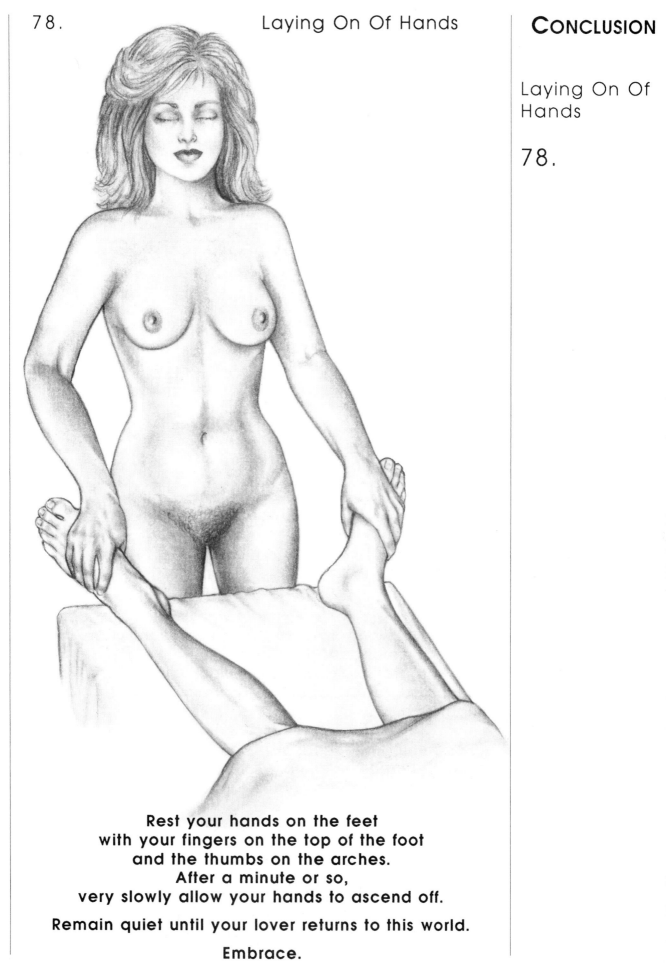

**Rest your hands on the feet
with your fingers on the top of the foot
and the thumbs on the arches.
After a minute or so,
very slowly allow your hands to ascend off.**

**Remain quiet until your lover returns to this world.**

**Embrace.**

# APPENDIX

## Eroticizing Safer-Sex

Massage in general
is considered in AIDS safer-sex guidelines
to be a no-risk or very-low-risk activity.

When there is uncertainty
about the giver's or receiver's health
or if either partner is communicable
with the AIDS virus,
you may wish to read the following.

Current research indicates that when
blood, ejaculate, or vaginal lubrications
come in contact
with a broken skin or membranous tissue surface,
the transmission risk may increase.

Should you prefer to follow AIDS safer-sex practices
when massaging the male or female genital area,
it is recommended
to wear latex or vinyl examination gloves,
which you can purchase at a pharmacy or surgical
supply store.

(Concerning infectious skin conditions,
such as herpes lesions or venereal warts,
it is recommended to entirely forego contact
with the communicable area
or to consult a medical professional.)

When using a latex product,
apply only a water-based lubricant
since oil can deteriorate latex.
If the water-based lubricant contains nonoxynol-9,
which can destroy the AIDS virus on contact,
the protection will be supplemented.
Some people, though, are sensitive to nonoxynol-9.

An alternative or an addition to wearing gloves
in a male genital massage
is to place a condom on the penis.
Try a few drops of water-based lubricant
in the tip of the condom before unrolling it.
Some of the strokes in this book, however,
are best suited for gloves without a condom.

At first, these protective measures
might appear as intrusions or hindrances.
After exploration, you may find,
as many others have,
that latex and vinyl examination gloves
provide some uniquely smooth sensations,
that the water-based lubricant inside the condom
creates heretofore unexperienced pleasures.

Eroticizing safer-sex means
letting go of expectations
and allowing the discovery of new worlds.
Giving the touch of love,
as in the sensual massage offered in this book,
can bring us all closer
to these new worlds of pleasure.

# Acknowledgments

The underlying massage style in *Erotic Massage* evolved in the early days of humanistic psychology. We wish to express our gratitude to Margaret Elke, whose work in massage and sensuality has influenced many, and to the pioneering teachers at Esalen Institute.

The students and faculty of The Institute for Advanced Study of Human Sexuality in San Francisco have continuously supported our teaching massage as a means to bring the sensual and intimate qualities into the sexual expression.

We are deeply indebted to Clark Taylor, Ph.D. and David Lourea, Ed.D. of the Sexologists' Sexual Health Project in San Francisco for their support in eroticizing safer-sex. We are equally thankful to Molly Hogan, R.N., Norma Wilcox, R.N., and Sharon Miller, M.S..

Finding an artist with both the sensitivity and the willingness to illustrate the subject matter of this book was a major undertaking. Then, drawing the illustrations was a major undertaking of time. We have nothing but praise for Kyle Spencer and hope this, her first book, is only the beginning of a successful career.

Our dear friend, Ellen Gunther, M.D., provided the photography on which the illustrations were based. She is such a joy.

This project could never have been accomplished without direct financial assistance from Al Ruiz, Carolyn Hardies, Christian Zangerle, Chuck Garrigues, Jim Everett, John Jaeger, Mary Campisi, Paul Johnson, Peter and Monika Riedl, and Yvon Dallaire.

We greatly appreciate help from so many others in so many ways: Al Schmid, Beau Lee, Betty Chase, Carl and Suzanne Miller, Ed Kammerman, Flavio Amorin, Jacques Lalanne, Jim Sensar, Joseph Kramer, John Robinson, Laura Takeshita, Lori Grace, Lynn Craig, Maria Silva, Mark Baltus, Mary Jane Harper, Nora LaCorte, A. Pat Malcolm, Sue Zimbauer, Tim Hancock, Wendell Lipscomb, as well as others.